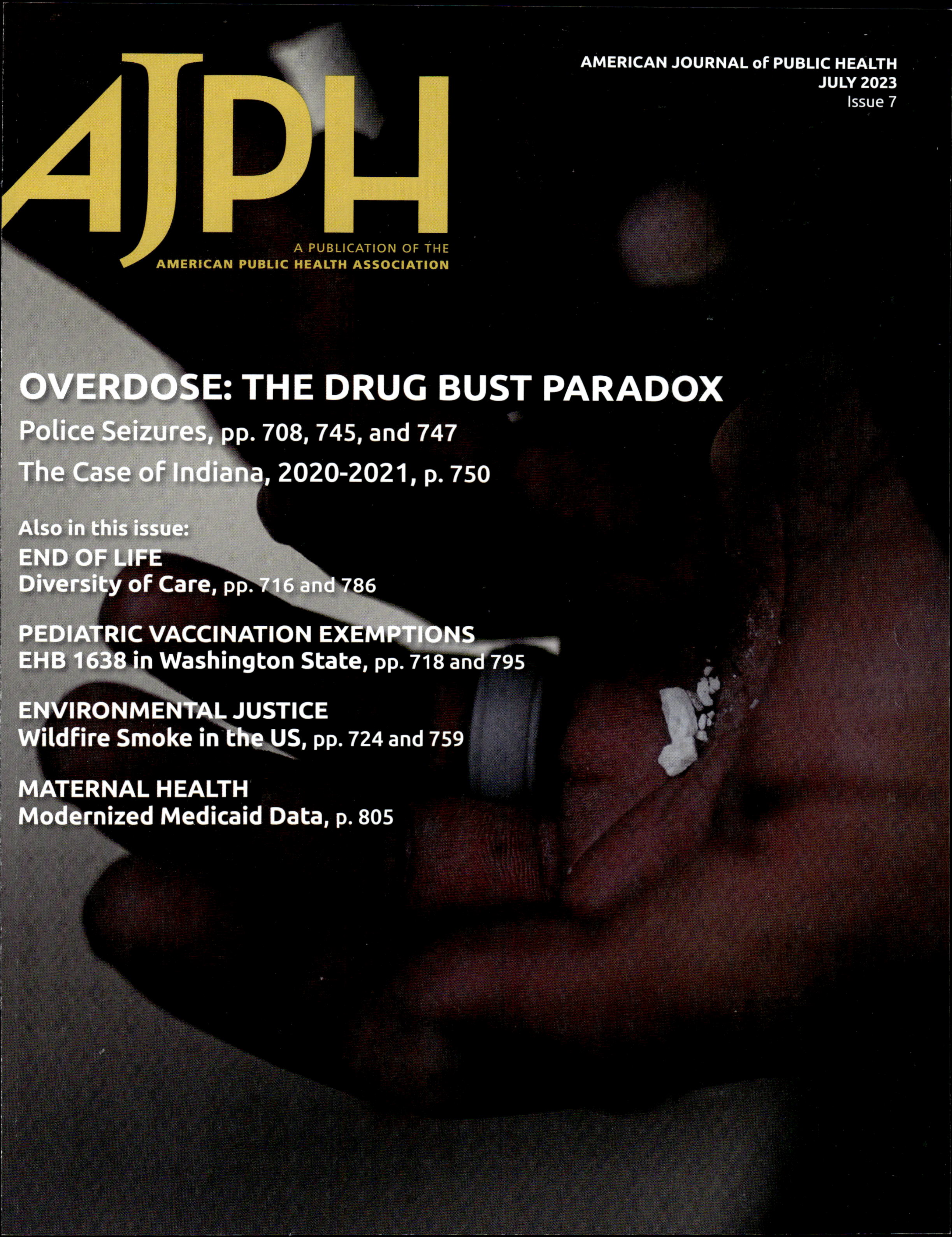

AJPH

A PUBLICATION OF THE
AMERICAN PUBLIC HEALTH ASSOCIATION

AMERICAN JOURNAL of PUBLIC HEALTH
JULY 2023
Issue 7

OVERDOSE: THE DRUG BUST PARADOX

Police Seizures, pp. 708, 745, and 747
The Case of Indiana, 2020-2021, p. 750

Also in this issue:

END OF LIFE
Diversity of Care, pp. 716 and 786

PEDIATRIC VACCINATION EXEMPTIONS
EHB 1638 in Washington State, pp. 718 and 795

ENVIRONMENTAL JUSTICE
Wildfire Smoke in the US, pp. 724 and 759

MATERNAL HEALTH
Modernized Medicaid Data, p. 805

APHA
AMERICAN PUBLIC HEALTH ASSOCIATION
For science. For action. For health.

AJPH®, published monthly, is the official Journal of the American Public Health Association®, 800 I St NW, Washington, DC 20001-3710; (202) 777- APHA; TDD (202) 777-2500. APHA is a nongovernmental professional society founded in 1872, representing all disciplines and specialties in public health.

The *American Journal of Public Health*® (*AJPH*) (print ISSN: 0090-0036; electronic ISSN: 1541- 0048), first published in 1911, is the official journal of the American Public Health Association® (APHA). The oldest and largest organization of public health professionals in the world, APHA represents approximately 30 000 members from more than 50 occupations of public health.

Submissions: Visit www.editorialmanager.com/ajph or ajph.edmgr.com for online manuscript preparation and submission guidelines. Contributions of original unpublished research, social science analyses, scholarly essays, critical commentaries, departments, and letters to the editor are welcome. Questions? Write ajph.submissions@apha.org or call APHA at (202) 777-2469.

Print plus online subscriptions: Institutional price (print copy with online access for a single institution and all authorized users, regardless of geographic location) varies by size of organization and ranges from $993–$1445 for US organizations, and $1073–$1526 for international organizations (air delivery); multiple campuses not permitted without special arrangement. Details of the tiered pricing system at https://subscriptionoffice.com/pages/apha-landing-page. To order, write apha.subscriptions@apha.org.

Online only subscriptions: Institutional price for one institution and its authorized users (regardless of geographic location) is $878–$1307. To order, write apha.subscriptions@apha.org. For academic consortia or multisite corporate subscriptions, contact apha.subscriptions@apha.org.

Print-only subscriptions: Institutional price is US $701, $782 international.

Back print issues: A limited number of print issues are for sale. Single copies are US $49, $55 international (air delivery). Shipping included; prepay only. To order, write apha.subscriptions@apha.org.

Reprints: For prices and ordering information on 50 or more reprints, check the Reprints section at www.ajph.org. To order smaller quantities of reprints (rush delivery), use the "Purchase Article" link on the article site itself.

Electronic access: Online articles more than 10 years old are available free for personal use at www.ajph.org. Recent articles are available through pay-per-view: single PDF article for $24, single issue access for 24 hours for $33, or entire site access for 24 hours for $38.

Postal information: Periodicals postage paid at Washington, DC, and additional mailing offices. Postmaster: Send address changes to American Journal of Public Health, 800 I St NW, Washington, DC 20001-3710.

Address changes: Send to AJPH, Membership Department (members) or AJPH Subscriptions (subscribers), APHA, 800 I St NW, Washington, DC 20001-3710. Or write to membership.mail@apha. org (members) or apha.subscriptions@apha.org (subscribers).

Advertising: For pricing and other information, see www.ajph.org. Please write to ashell.alston@apha.org or call (202) 777-2470 for other advertising opportunities. Ask about special exhibit packages and sponsorships. Acceptance of advertising by the *Journal* does not imply endorsement of products.

Indexes: Publications that index or abstract articles from AJPH include the following: Ageline, Assia (Applied Social Science Index and Abstracts), Biological Abstracts, Chemical Abstracts, CINAHL, Criminal Justice Abstracts, EMBASE, EMCare, Environmental Abstracts, e-psyche, ERIC, ETOH (Alcohol and Alcohol Problems Science Database), Excerpta Medica, Food Science and Technology, General Science Index, Grateful Med, Hospital Literature Index, Human Resources Abstracts, International Pharmaceutical Abstracts (IPA), Medline, Physical Education Index, Pollution Abstracts, Psychological Abstracts, PsychINFO, Safety Science Abstracts, Sage Family Studies Abstracts, Sage Human Resources Abstracts, Science Citation Index, SCOPUS, SIIC Data Bases, Social Work Research and Abstracts, and Statistical Reference Index (SRI)/LexisNexis.

Medscape Publishers' Circle

AJPH

A PUBLICATION OF THE
AMERICAN PUBLIC HEALTH ASSOCIATION

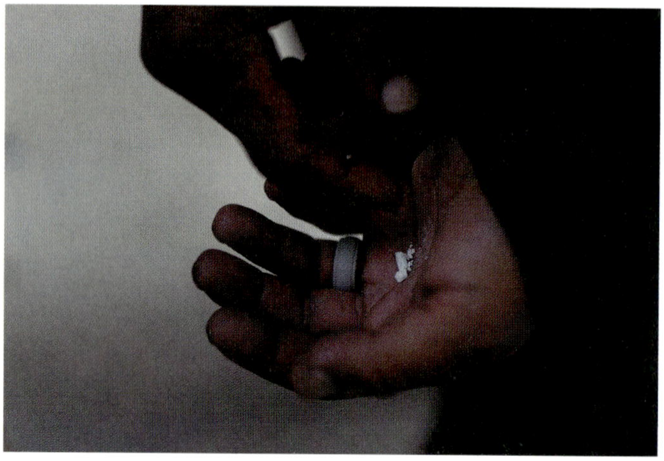

COVER: Person holding pieces of fentanyl. Use of this powerful synthetic opioid, which is cheap to produce and is often sold as is or laced in other drugs, has exploded. Because it is 50 times more potent than heroin, even a small dose can be fatal. It has quickly become the deadliest drug in the nation, according to the US Drug Enforcement Administration.

Cover concept and selection by Aleisha Kropf. Photo by Jae C. Hong/AP Images. Printed with permission.

APHA
AMERICAN PUBLIC HEALTH ASSOCIATION
For science. For action. For health.

Promoting public health research, policy, practice, and education is the *AJPH* mission. As we widen our scope to embrace global issues, we also sharpen our focus to support the needs of public health practitioners. We invite contributions of original unpublished research, opinion and commentary, and letters to the editor.

The *Journal* is printed on acid-free recycled paper.

OPEN ACCESS ONLINE ONLY PODCAST DATA SUPPLEMENT AVAILABLE

EDITOR'S CHOICE

708 We Can't Arrest Our Way Out of Overdose: The Drug Bust Paradox
N. Dasgupta

BOOKS & MEDIA

709 A Revolution Betrayed: A History of Tobacco Smoking and Public Health in the USSR
A. Morabia

713 The COVID-19 Vaccination Story: Public Health Expertise Is as Vital as Private-Sector Ingenuity
R. Hughes IV

OPINIONS, IDEAS, & PRACTICE

EDITORIALS

716 Diversity of End-of-Life Care in the Boom of Deaths at Old Age
Q. Feng

718 To EHB 1638 or Not to EHB 1638? For Immunization Policymakers, That Is the Question
J. T. B. Williams and S. T. O'Leary

721 Probability Samples Provide a Means of Benchmarking and Adjusting for Data Collected From Nonprobability Samples
M. R. Elliott

724 It's the Smoke, Not the Fire
D. P. Eisenman

726 Mortality Inequities: Power, Theory, and Data Considerations
J. L. Jahn and S. M. Hernandez

729 An Equity-Focused Care Continuum Framework for Mpox and Future Infectious Disease Outbreaks: A Public Health of Consequence, July 2023
R. A. Pitts, A. Cifuentes Kottkamp, and O. Mgbako

732 Looking Back: Decarcerating Immigration Prisons as a Tool for Improved Health
C. Patler, A. Saadi, and A. Arulanantham

736 Looking Back: How the COVID-19 Pandemic Provided Opportunity to Equitably Improve Meal Provision
C. R. Singleton and G. M. McLoughlin

PERSPECTIVES

739 How Green Spaces Can Combat Gun Violence in America
J. E. Dobbs and J. V. Sakran

742 Veteran Truckers, the Supply Chain, and the Metabolic Syndrome: A Convergence of Crises
M. A. Dunn, E. B. Tapper, and S. S. Rogal

LAW ENFORCEMENT DRUG MARKET DISRUPTIONS ON OVERDOSE

745 Police Drug Seizures Cannot Solve the Problem of Toxic Drug Supply in North America
P. Dietze

747 At the Crossroads in the Opioid Overdose Epidemic: Will Evidence-Based "Radical" but Rational Drug Policy Strategies Prevail?
G. J. Stahler, J. Mennis, and S. Belenko

RESEARCH & ANALYSIS

LAW ENFORCEMENT DRUG MARKET DISRUPTIONS ON OVERDOSE

750 Spatiotemporal Analysis Exploring the Effect of Law Enforcement Drug Market Disruptions on Overdose, Indianapolis, Indiana, 2020–2021
B. Ray, S. J. Korzeniewski, G. Mohler, J. J. Carroll, B. del Pozo, G. Victor, P. Huynh, and B. J. Hedden

CLIMATE CHANGE

759 Social Vulnerability in US Communities Affected by Wildfire Smoke, 2011 to 2021
J. Vargo, B. Lappe, M. C. Mirabelli, and K. C. Conlon

METHODS

768 Stratified Simple Random Sampling Versus Volunteer Community-Wide Sampling for Estimates of COVID-19 Prevalence
R. J. Keith, R. H. Holm, A. R. Amraotkar, M. M. Bezold, J. M. Brick, A. M. Bushau-Sprinkle, K. T. Hamorsky, K. T. Kitterman, K. E. Palmer, T. Smith, R. Yeager, and A. Bhatnagar

778 Public Health Impacts of Vaccines for COVID-19 and Beyond: Opportunities to Overcome Technical and Regulatory Barriers for Randomized Trials
L. Kennedy-Shaffer

OPEN-THEMED RESEARCH

786 Variation in End-of-Life Trajectories in Persons Aged 70 Years and Older, Sweden, 2018–2020
M. Ebeling, A. C. Meyer, and K. Modig

795 State Policy Removing the Personal Belief Exemption for Measles, Mumps, and Rubella (MMR) School Immunization Requirement, Washington State, 2014–2022
T. P. Moore, J. C. Bennett, K. Graff, M. Rao, O. Augusto, H. Y. Chu, B. H. Wagenaar, and T. R. Bell

805 Using Modernized Medicaid Data to Advance Evidence-Based Improvements in Maternal Health
J. R. Daw, S. G. Auty, L. K. Admon, and S. H. Gordon

811 Examining Smoking Prevalence Disparities in Virginia Counties by Rurality, Appalachian Status, and Social Vulnerability, 2011–2019
A. Pilehvari, W. You, R. A. Krukowski, and M. A. Little

815 Evaluation of Public Health Contact Tracing for Mpox Among Gay, Bisexual, and Other Men Who Have Sex With Men—10 US Jurisdictions, May 17–July 31, 2022
A. B. Cope, R. D. Kirkcaldy, P. J. Weidle, D. A. Jackson, N. Laramee, R. Weber, J. Rowse, A. Mangla, B. Fox, K. E. Saunders, K. Taniguchi, L. Usagawa, M. E. Cahill, P. Harrington, E. K. Ricketts, K. Harbi, L. Malec, T. G. Templin, D. Drociuk, T. Hannibal, R. Klos, and K. T. Bernstein

BACKMATTER

OTHER DEPARTMENTS

824 Subscription Form

AJPH July 2023, Vol 113, No. 7

We Can't Arrest Our Way Out of Overdose: The Drug Bust Paradox

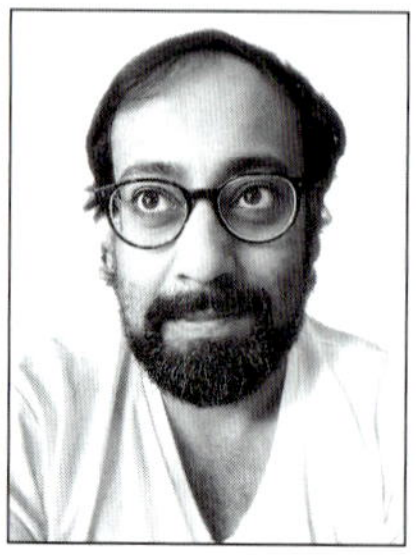

In speaking with police about preventing overdose, the officers' common refrain is "We aren't going to arrest our way out of this" (https://bit.ly/3O3d4Vc). And among public health practitioners, there is weariness that our best efforts have not yet stemmed the tide of overdose deaths. In this context, an article in this issue of *AJPH* lends credence to law enforcement's mantra and provides health policymakers with evidence to take bolder action.

In this issue of *AJPH*, Ray et al. (p. 750) explored whether overdose increased or decreased in proximity to drug arrests in Indianapolis, Indiana. They found that within a six-minute walk (500 m) of each drug arrest, opioid overdose deaths doubled. Elevated fatal and nonfatal opioid overdoses were sustained over one, two, and three weeks.

What could explain this remarkable finding? In an editorial in this issue of *AJPH*, Dietze (p. 745), drawing on experience from Australia, explores possible causal mechanisms related to interrupted opioid tolerance, which leaves people at higher risk for overdose when the same quantity is used after a period of abstinence. Correspondingly, Ray et al. did not find the same association with stimulants, which are not subject to the same discontinuation immediate overdose risk. Conceptualizing stimulants as a control group, and employing a counterfactual modeling strategy, provides a counterpoint to criticism that increasing drug arrests are only a parallel association with increasing overdoses.

Alternatively, interruption of supply drives people to new drug suppliers, who may have levels of active ingredient to which the individual is unaccustomed. Further investigations are needed to evaluate these ecological findings in causal inference frameworks.

Because of the importance of the findings and specialized methods, *AJPH* put the article through an extensive peer review process, with eight independent reviewers, who included legal scholars, epidemiologists, and geospatial statisticians, as well as internal statistical and methodological reviews by editors. The supplementary material includes additional data that were requested during review, including quantities of drugs seized.

We also invited the leadership of the Indianapolis Metropolitan Police Department (IMPD) to comment because they provided the data. Unfortunately, their duties could not accommodate our publication schedule. We welcome letters from the IMPD and other law enforcement agencies. We commend the IMPD for participating in this scientific inquiry because the policy questions have weighty importance. This study demonstrates that law enforcement data have applications in answering difficult public health questions.

Other forms of police data remain siloed. Currently, we find out what is in street drugs only when it is too late: crime labs after arrest or autopsy after overdose. Recently the *Los Angeles Times* revealed that law enforcement in Los Angeles, California, may have failed to inform public health authorities about an emerging dangerous fentanyl adulterant (xylazine) for four years (https://bit.ly/3VYYlak). The adulterant has been implicated in increased overdoses and the emergence of disfiguring skin ulcers. Those four years could have been used to develop education, prevention, and treatment.

These examples call into question whether US policing, as it currently stands, is a reliable agent of drug harm prevention. There is growing scientific evidence to support what many on the street already know: the narrow mission of law enforcement may exacerbate drug harms. Over the past decade, there has been a gradual ideological shift in law enforcement training, away from military-style "enforcers" and toward "guardians" of communities focused on crisis intervention and greater attention to social interactions (https://bit.ly/42LttSb).

Back in Los Angeles, in response to the earlier criticism, the sheriff's department agreed to track xylazine in seized drugs and left open the door to update their detection methods if the information is helpful. With proper evidence and public health impetus, it is possible for some law enforcement agencies to change course (https://bit.ly/3nQl1Cn).

Ray et al. also provide useful metrics of law enforcement's expected reach. In a city with a population of one million, there were seven drug seizures per day. By comparison, there were 17.2 nonfatal overdoses recorded by emergency medical services and 1.6 fatal overdoses. There are almost three times more overdoses than there are police interventions to seize drugs. Even with a predominantly law enforcement approach, interdiction is grossly outmatched. This lends credence to the refrain that we aren't going to arrest our way out of this.

On the maps of Indianapolis, no one can be surprised that drug arrests are overrepresented in neighborhoods with lower financial resources and those with more racialized minority residents. Considering the finding that drug arrests may exacerbate overdose mortality, disproportionate policing of Black neighborhoods deserves renewed investigation, as overdose death rates in this demographic are now the highest (https://bit.ly/3BffcS5).

As a nation, our drug policies are collectively not working. Fleming et al. have noted the public health funding paradox, whereby taxpayers are simultaneously subsidizing separate government policies that prevent and exacerbate the same problem (https://bit.ly/3I4WnEJ). In an editorial in this issue of *AJPH*, Stahler et al. (p. 747) contextualize the findings in evidence-based interventions. To address the very real concerns from both law enforcement and public health practitioners, it is time to find new solutions. AJPH

Nabarun Dasgupta, PhD, MPH
AJPH Associate Editor

DOI: https://doi.org/10.2105/AJPH.2023.307329

54 Years Ago

Concerning Heroin Use and Official Records

"The present paper . . . takes exception to the view that all addicts ultimately come to police attention. It presents in support of its position several case histories of individuals in street drug use who mainlined heroin in heavy dosages over long periods of time. These subjects conceived of themselves as addicts . . . but remained, according to their personal testimony and our search of the records, unknown to either law enforcement or hospital authorities as being involved with drugs. . . . [W]e found our subjects with little difficulty, and . . . they maintained that they were aware of others of their kind. By no means would we suggest that their numbers are sizable. But we feel it important to document their existence because epidemiological information, upon which public health policies regarding drug use may be founded, should take into account the existence of undetected heroin addiction, as well as the polemic corollary of this fact which maintains that, absent criminal and civil commitment statutes, individuals may well be able to perform adequately while using opiates, particularly if the drugs are cheap and accessible."

From AJPH, *October 1969, p. 1888*

109 Years Ago

Drug Addictions, A Public Health Problem

[I]t may seem a strong statement to make that over 50 per cent of drug users owe their habit to the medical profession, and yet I am convinced that my figures are not far wrong. . . . In many instances these first doses were not give at the bedside to allay severe pain, but handed out to office patients with apparently as little concern as a dose of calomel. Codeine, morphine, heroin and laudanum are all thus passed over to the temporary sufferer; the neurotic woman with obscure symptoms, the young mechanic with a broken arm, the over-tired businessman; to young and old, it matters not, who chance to stray into the wrong office and who pay the price of their evil choice years after their faces are forgotten and their fees spent by the "expert" who so readily relieved their symptoms. Not only are these drugs carelessly prescribed but we find many repeated orders to "refill the prescription and then let me hear from you," the patient in entire ignorance, not infrequently learning for the first time from another physician or a conscientious druggist the nature of the "remedy" in which they have been placing their hope of cure."

From AJPH, *January 1914, pp. 32–33*

A Revolution Betrayed: A History of Tobacco Smoking and Public Health in the USSR

Alfredo Morabia, MD, PhD

ABOUT THE AUTHOR

Alfredo Morabia is Editor-in-Chief of AJPH *and is with City University of New York and Columbia University, New York, NY.*

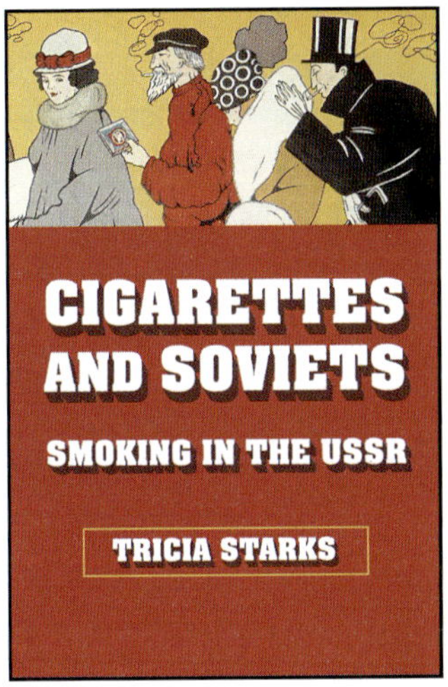

Cigarettes and Soviets: Smoking in the USSR (NIU Series in Slavic, East European, and Eurasian Studies)
By Tricia Starks
DeKalb, IL: Northern Illinois University Press; 2022
Hardcover: 324 pp.; $44.95
ISBN-13: 978-1501765483

This new book by Tricia Starks makes two important and original contributions to the existing public health literature: it recounts an episode of the history of tobacco different from the much more studied one in the West, and it is the liveliest history I know of the evolution of public health in the USSR.

The book's nine chapters, between the introduction ("The Revolutionary Soviet Smoker") and the epilogue ("The Post-Soviet Smoker"), have titles (in quotes in this paragraph) that characterize the evolving relation of tobacco to Soviet society across the century: tobacco production and consumption was "Attacked" immediately after the October Revolution of 1917 by Commissar Semashko, who aimed for tobacco prohibition; it was "Resurrected" after 1917 when factories were nationalized and revitalized; and it was "Sold" thanks to revolutionary advertising that boosted communist consumption. Still, tobacco addiction was "Treated" in specialized dispensaries, with 40% to 50% success in 1928 (p. 93). The antitobacco revolutionary goals were "Unfulfilled" under Stalin. Tobacco was "Mobilized" during World War II. After 1945, tobacco was "Recovered" from war's destruction, produced by women, and consumed by men. It later was "Partnered" with Western tobacco companies in the 1950s and 1960s and, finally, "Pressured" by public health in the 1980s and after.

BOLSHEVIK PUBLIC HEALTH

Starks is a professor of history at the Fulbright College of Arts and Sciences at the University of Arkansas. Her previous books already focused on the intersection of culture and public health in the Russian and Soviet contexts. *The Body Soviet: Propaganda, Hygiene, and the Revolutionary State* (The University of Wisconsin Press, 2009) was about the concept of hygiene and health developed by the Bolsheviks. *Smoking Under the Tsars: A History of Tobacco in Imperial Russia* (Cornell University Press, 2018) covers, as the title clearly states, the history of tobacco before the Russian Revolution.[1] *Cigarettes and Soviets* begins with the 1917 Bolshevik Revolution, which took place in a population already heavily addicted to a form of rolled cigarette with high nicotine content called *papyrosa*.

The Bolsheviks promoted reasons and ways to oppose tobacco that differed from those to come in the West. Smoking was tied to capitalism, and it was expected that the social and cultural revolution would defeat tobacco. The tool was public health:

> The Bolshevik seizure of power created opportunities for the maintenance of public health . . . animosity to tobacco stemmed from the mass imposition of its smell and an opinion among some revolutionary-era doctors that nicotine was a poison that attacked the nervous system. (p. 5)

Vladimir I. Lenin, one of the two main leaders of the Bolshevik party, and the

Health Commissar, equivalent to a minister of health, Nikolai Semashko, attempted to curtail the production and the imports of tobacco. They failed. The income from state taxes on tobacco sales was too important. On the other hand, they launched an ambitious public health campaign to discourage new smokers and encourage smokers to stop smoking:

> Semashko waged a war against tobacco unprecedented for its intended scope and exceptional in range, making the Soviets the first country in the world, in 1920, to entertain a national health program to curtail tobacco production, sales, imports, exports, and use with the goal of eventually stamping out tobacco. (p. 2)

An important aspect of this campaign when compared with other early 20th century antitobacco attitudes is that it was real, objectified by the numbers of clinics, posters, and articles available:

> Pamphlets, posters, slogans, and lectures flooded the population with information on how to live, work, and rest. Museums, banners, and sandwich boards surrounded urban dwellers while trains, boats, and traveling displays toured the countryside. Workers' clubs staged lectures, films, slide shows, and agitation plays with new lifestyle messages. (p. 17)

The Commissariat for Public Health (Narkomzdrav) developed a massive, creative propaganda campaign aimed to promote a new Soviet man, woman, and child, free of tobacco addiction (p. 31). Semashko did not achieve his full ideal, but the USSR established the earliest national antitobacco campaigns and funded public cessation clinics.

STALINIST PUBLIC HEALTH

This prevention campaign was interrupted when Stalin and his followers, in the years following Lenin's death in 1924, dominated the party and the Soviet state. Cigarettes became a component of the support and awards for increased productivity of industrial and rural workers. Leon Trotsky described Stalinism as a betrayal of the socialist goals of the October Revolution of 1917.[2] He did not mention public health, but in the sphere of tobacco consumption, Stalinism corresponded to a betrayal of the public health Semashko had attempted to develop.

In 1931, Anastas Ivanovich Mikoian, from the People's Commissariat of the food industry, praised tobacco workers for fueling the Stalinist industrialization drive, boasting that the Soviet tobacco industry had been successfully Stalinized and that its production volume would "occupy the second place in the world behind the United States" (p. 119). As Starks puts it, "cessation had been sacrificed on the altar of steel" (p. 135).

During World War II, tobacco and cigarettes became an essential staple for the armies, on both the Nazi and Soviet sides. Entire cigarette factories were moved away from the front to maintain production. Tobacco fields became coveted targets of the Nazi conquest or of the Soviet resistance.

CIGARETTES AND SPUTNIKS

The USSR emerged from World War II with dire tobacco addiction levels. Moreover, the country had lost an estimated 28 million citizens and soldiers. The men-to-women ratio had dropped. The public health impact of tobacco was observable, but the wave of antitobacco policies in Western societies of the 1960s and after did not reach Eastern Europe. Cigarettes were advertised by the state and linked to the space conquest (Figure 1). American and British tobacco corporations seized the opportunity to penetrate and control the Soviet market, using coproduction of Soviet brands or selling their own brands (e.g., Marlboro).

Finally, in the 1980s, the public health reaction to tobacco began in the USSR, paradoxically returning to the original intentions of Lenin and Semashko. Today, the smell of tobacco that used to characterize the Russian and Soviet societies seems to have largely disappeared. Smoking is restricted to delimited spaces, as Lenin used to do when he forced smokers to apply for their turn to go and smoke in the restrooms during the meetings of the party.

A BEAUTIFUL BOOK

Starks has written a literally beautiful book, full of illustrations of tobacco packs and advertisement posters over a century. I read the book once as a pdf without the images, then as a pdf with images, and finally was able to read with delight the hardcover version. The illustrations are esthetically compelling, and Starks excels in describing their content, hidden meaning, and even taste and feel for the smoker. Here is, for example, Starks's comment about Figure 1 (which I chose because Starks owns the copyright):

> The optimism of the painting shines through in the joyous coloring and lovingly detailed spacecraft. The ten packs arrayed flat within the carton display a blue sphere on a white background against which the docking crafts are framed [Figure 1].

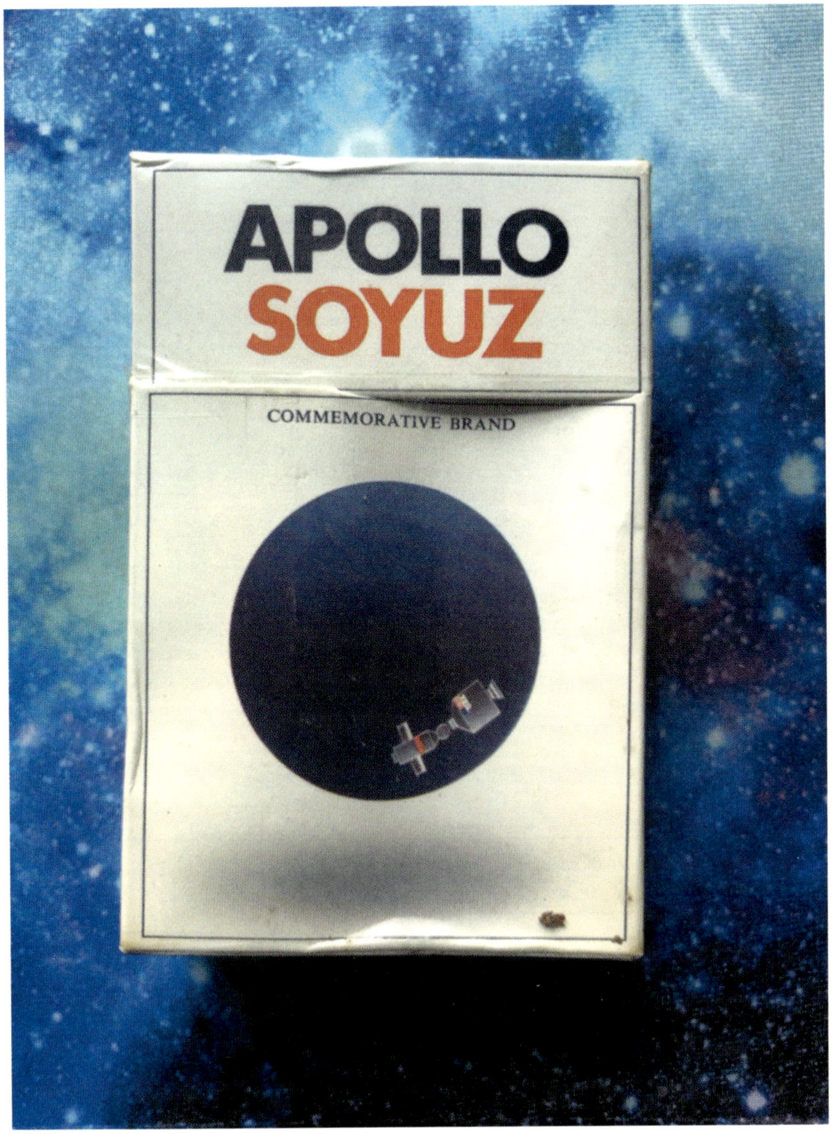

FIGURE 1— Photo: Pack of Apollo-Soyuz, 1975.

Source. Tricia Starks's collection. Printed with permission.

> In block, sans serif lettering Soiuz-Apollon or Apollo-Soyuz adorned the top of the pack in red and blue with Russian on one side and English the other. The cigarette itself had American-made cellulose acetate filters with cork tipping and blue lettering on brilliant white cigarette paper. The feel of the packaging was as pleasing and modern as the look. Silver foil lined the inside of the box. A six-millimeter red tape could remove the covering cellophane while also popping out the first smoke. Compared to American products, the cigarettes were a bit heavier with lower nicotine (1.2 mg), higher sugar, and twenty mg of tar. (p. 184–185)

I feel challenged to find weaknesses in the book. I can mention two minor ones. There is an imbalance in the historical coverage: the two strongest parts are the history of tobacco use in the early Bolshevik and Stalinist period (1917–1956) and the illustrations. The more recent history of tobacco in the last years of the USSR and current Russia is less systematically covered. A second comment is even more subtle. The title refers to Soviets, which evokes the workers and people's councils that were intended to allow the masses to weigh in on the local, district, and national policy. However, the book suggests that most of the public health attempts to control tobacco consumption were top-down governmental decisions. A discussion of the role of the Soviets in these policy decisions would have been of great interest.

Overall, Starks takes us on a voyage in Soviet public health, revealing, beyond smoking, what was the daily life of its population over the 20th century. Because it enriches the pool of unique cases of tobacco policy in the history of public health, *Cigarettes and Soviets* does something analogous to what Anatole Kopp's *Town and Revolution: Soviet Architecture and City Planning, 1917–1935* did for architecture. Kopp incorporated the Soviet architectural avant-garde of the 1920s into general historiography. He showed that Soviet architecture was not a relic from the past but a working method that failed for very precise economic, political, and cultural reasons.[3(p14)] Similarly, Starks has now incorporated the legacy of early Soviet public health policy and practice into the tobacco historiography.

Starks's style is clear, engaging, and often witty. I recommend *Cigarettes and Soviets* to anyone interested in the history of tobacco, the history of public health, and the history of the USSR. AJPH

CORRESPONDENCE

Correspondence should be sent to Alfredo Morabia, MD, PhD, Barry Commoner Center for Health and the Environment, Queens College,

CUNY, 65-30 Kissena Blvd, Flushing, NY 11367 (e-mail: amorabia@qc.cuny.edu). Reprints can be ordered at https://ajph.org by clicking the "Reprints" link.

PUBLICATION INFORMATION

Full Citation: Morabia A. A revolution betrayed: a history of tobacco smoking and public health in the USSR. *Am J Public Health*. 2023;113(7): 709–712.

Acceptance Date: March 24, 2023.

DOI: https://doi.org/10.2105/AJPH.2023.307307

ACKNOWLEDGMENTS

I thank Daniel M. Fox and Michael C. Costanza for comments and edits on an earlier version of this article.

CONFLICTS OF INTEREST

The author has no conflicts of interest to disclose.

REFERENCES

1. Morabia A. Anti-tobacco propaganda: Soviet Union versus Nazi Germany. *Am J Public Health*. 2017; 107(11):1708–1710. https://doi.org/10.2105/AJPH.2017.304087
2. Trotsky L. *The Revolution Betrayed. What Is the Soviet Union and Where Is It Going? [1936]*. New York, NY: Pathfinder Press; 1973.
3. Yakushenko O. Anatole Kopp's town and revolution as history and a manifesto: a reactualization of Russian constructivism in the West in the 1960s. *J Art Historiogr*. 2016;14. Available at: https://hdl.handle.net/1814/71644. Accessed March 28, 2022.

The COVID-19 Vaccination Story: Public Health Expertise Is as Vital as Private-Sector Ingenuity

Richard Hughes IV, JD, MPH

ABOUT THE AUTHOR

Richard Hughes is a partner with Epstein Becker Green, Washington, DC, and a professorial lecturer in law at The George Washington University Law School, Washington, DC.

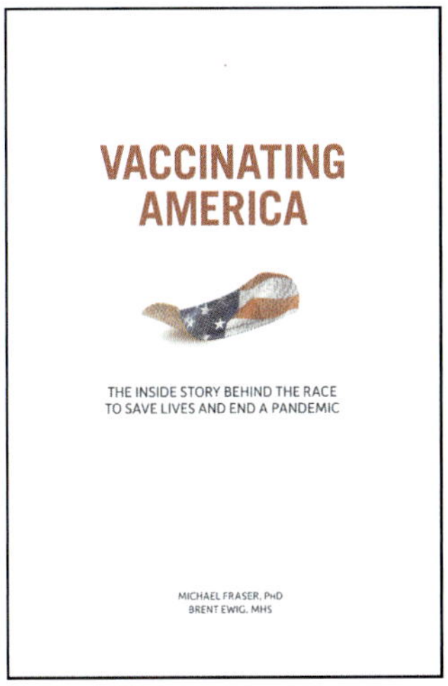

Vaccinating America: The Inside Story Behind the Race to Save Lives and End a Pandemic
By Michael Fraser and Brent Ewig
Washington, DC: APHA Press; 2022
Paperback: 250 pp; $55.00
ISBN-10: 0875533329
ISBN-13: 978-0875533322

The COVID-19 pandemic response enlisted the efforts and resources of a multitude of federal, state, and local agencies, as well as private-sector entities that developed and manufactured vaccines, therapies, masks, and ventilators. A successful response to COVID-19 would not have been possible without both a whole-of-government effort and private-sector ingenuity. While the response was not always smooth, the public and private sectors came together to deliver more than 200 million vaccines, sparing more than 2.2 million lives, averting more than 17 million hospitalizations, and saving almost $1 trillion health care dollars. Yet, recent research has shown that public trust in public health during the COVID-19 response was not especially high, suggesting, perhaps, that its efforts were not well understood.[1]

Vaccinating America: The Inside Story Behind the Race to Save Lives and End a Pandemic by Michael Fraser, PhD, MS, and Brent Ewig, MHS, provides an unparalleled perspective of the greatest public health undertaking in perhaps a generation. It is at once objective and thorough in addressing all sides of the vaccination effort while also providing the reader with a unique public health vantage point.

IN THE ARENA

Both Fraser and Ewig have extensive experience working with state and local public health agencies and have devoted their careers to advancing the nation's public health. Their knowledge and perspective come through strongly throughout the book.

Fraser is the current CEO of the Association of State and Territorial Health Officials (ASTHO). His organization represents and supports state health officers (SHOs) and their staffs across the country. SHOs are at the helm of state health agencies, which work to protect, promote, and advance public health every day. These agencies run myriad public health programs with the support of a dedicated, often undercompensated workforce.

When a disease outbreak on any scale occurs in their jurisdiction, SHOs bear the responsibility of advising the governors who appointed them, evaluating the epidemiology to understand the scope of the threat, and instituting policies to protect the public from that threat. This is typically done in close collaboration across state, local, and federal governments under an emergency response posture to facilitate rapid decision-making and implementation. SHOs operate in a realm that demands political and public accountability as they strive to do what is best for their citizens. Thus, they often bear the brunt of public backlash over public health measures and have even been subjected to death threats.

Ewig is both a former ASTHO staffer and the chief policy and government relations officer at the Association of Immunization Managers (AIM). AIM represents the leaders within state health agencies responsible for immunization programs. Most support for these programs comes to states through the Centers for Disease Control and Prevention (CDC) in the form of the Vaccines for Children program and Section 317 grant funding to support infrastructure and limited additional vaccine purchase. By and large, states provide little in the way of additional financial support to these programs, but it is these programs that bore the responsibility of ensuring that once COVID-19 vaccines reached their states' borders they made it the "last mile" and into arms.

It is from their deep experience working with these state officials, along with 20 in-depth supplemental interviews with revered vaccine and public health experts, that Fraser and Ewig were able to tell an insider's COVID-19 vaccination story. It is a story that the public would not otherwise hear but sorely needs to.

THE COVID-19 STORY THAT NEEDED TELLING

Vaccinating America begins by recounting the early days of the pandemic, which is familiar to the general public. Against the backdrop of fear and uncertainty, fueled by conspiracy theories perpetuated by the president of the United States, state health officials had to make important decisions about how to protect their citizens. Confusion reigned over which level and parts of government were in charge as some persistently denied that COVID-19 was a threat at all. This, in many ways, united the general public in the urgent desire for a vaccine.

The authors provide the all-important context of pre–COVID-19 underfunding, the lessons learned from previous pandemics, and President Bush's post-9/11 realization of the threat a future pandemic could pose to our country. The 2005 Pandemic Influenza Plan that was intended to guide our nation's response was largely ignored with respect to how information was communicated to the public and how vaccines would be distributed. This manifested in inconsistent information, jockeying of experts and spokespeople at the White House, and early stated intentions to rely on the military to distribute vaccines.

Public health professionals at the federal and state level were largely ignored from the beginning. The CDC was marginalized—its leaders' advice frequently rebuffed and its deep capabilities to work with states to successfully deliver vaccines overlooked.

Fraser and Ewig observe from an interview with former Massachusetts SHO John Auerbach that public health professionals not only understand the logistics of distributing vaccines, but they also know their communities and how to foster the much-needed public trust to run a successful vaccination campaign. Yet, the administration sadly omitted these professionals from planning efforts and even ignored their advice and offers of support and cooperation.

Eventually, of course, the federal government would gravitate toward reliance on the existing, well-established infrastructure of the CDC and state and local public health. But its efforts to engage those in charge of that infrastructure came far too late. So did the resources. The authors note that of the $30 billion the Trump administration had spent on Operation Warp Speed (OWS) before leaving office, state and territorial health departments were initially awarded a mere $200 million. An additional $140 million would arrive on the eve of the vaccine rollout. Compare those figures with the $8.4 billion a coalition of public health associations estimated would be needed to successfully carry out the vaccination campaign.

Ultimately, after all of the Trump administration's talk of militarized logistics, the CDC's distribution plan was followed. Channels and systems ordinarily used for public vaccine distribution were relied on by states. And state health officials bore the responsibility for onboarding all of the additional health care providers needed to vaccinate the masses, ordering and allocating vaccine product according to implementation phases, ensuring that vaccination sites were equipped with ultra-cold storage capabilities to safely receive and maintain vaccine doses, and managing data collection through a new federal system in addition to their own immunization information systems.

Before the rollout would begin, the Trump administration would create alarm by setting unexplained readiness dates in the run-up to the November 2020 election. And in the latest stages of planning, OWS leaders would once again rebuff outreach from public health officials, insisting they were too busy and could not entertain adding regular touch-points to their "already full calendars."

Once the vaccine rollout began, state health officials bore the blame of slow movement through the phased allocation of doses despite being hampered by a lack of federal guidance and then swift allocation changes. As public demand for vaccines faded into hesitancy and fatigue while variants caused surges, these same officials were responsible for encouraging the public in pursuit of optimal vaccination targets.

The authors provide important context on the origins of vaccine hesitancy and structural racism in the general and Black and Hispanic populations. As they observe from evidence, the right messenger—usually public health officials and an individual's own physician—can make all the difference. Politicization following the 2020 election and January 6, 2021, insurrection, with many Republican elected officials openly denying COVID-19 and vaccine science, only exacerbates the challenges of fostering public trust in vaccines.

LESSONS LEARNED

The authors conclude by identifying lessons that should be learned from the COVID-19 pandemic and applied during the next pandemic.

Funding Matters

On a normal day, state health agencies and their immunization programs are underresourced. A public health emergency might engender a moment of notice by lawmakers that leads to supplemental funding. But emergencies are fleeting. And so it goes as our nation's public health officials do their work on a shoestring budget with an expectation that they be prepared for the next pandemic. As the authors quote Claire Hannan, executive director of AIM, "expecting a robust public health response without adequate funding to support it is like creating a 'wishlist'" (p. 192).

Trust Matters

The authors suggest a two-pronged strategy for building needed public confidence in vaccines: (1) building off of strategies for messaging that resonates with communities of color, they suggest delivery by trusted messengers, and (2) holding content creators and social media platforms accountable for misinformation that erodes public confidence in vaccines. As they observe, all of the responsibility for accomplishing this strategy cannot fall to public health, but requires health care providers to step up and address misinformation on a "massive scale."

Local, National, and Global Action Matters

Even in a global pandemic, the authors observe the maxim that "all disasters are local." It is ironic that a Republican administration would need reminding that "no one-sized-fits-all plan would ever work for every community in America." But dedicated state and local public health officials were able to tailor federal guidance to work for their communities and deliver vaccines to the most rural reaches of our country, including remote Alaskan villages and territorial islands. The authors' perspective is that both local response and global intervention are needed to stop a disease.

Nonpartisanship Matters

Vaccination became a political pawn during the pandemic, immersing us in a strange twilight zone where the president and his supporters boasted that he delivered the lifesaving vaccine while simultaneously downplaying COVID-19's threat and suggesting that the scientific establishment was delaying the vaccine until after his election defeat. And, today, the American public is deeply divided over the COVID-19 vaccine along partisan lines. One cannot read *Vaccinating America* without feeling that trust in science and public health is an unfortunate victim of the pandemic.

Leadership Matters

The authors praise the successful leadership and outcomes of OWS and note that it should be celebrated along with the leadership of thousands of state and local public health professionals. This and any future vaccination campaign requires, they note, "setting a vision, bringing people together around a common goal achieving clarity of purpose and motivating others to achieve it" (p. 200).

CONCLUSION

In *Vaccinating America,* Fraser and Ewig underscore the importance of leadership at every level of government during a public health emergency, and we can hope it motivates our nation to better achieve it during the next pandemic. It is also the only book to date that provides a straightforward account of the governmental public health response to COVID-19.

Moreover, *Vaccinating America* should convince the reader that the expertise and efforts of public health were just as vital during the pandemic as the private-sector ingenuity that is more widely known and lauded. AJPH

CORRESPONDENCE

Correspondence should be sent to Richard Hughes IV, JD, MPH, 1227 25th St NW, Suite 700, Washington, DC 20037 (e-mail: rhughesiv@law.gwu.edu). Reprints can be ordered at https://ajph.org by clicking the "Reprints" link.

PUBLICATION INFORMATION

Full Citation: Hughes R. The COVID-19 vaccination story: public health expertise is as vital as private-sector ingenuity. *Am J Public Health*. 2023; 113(7):713–715.

Acceptance Date: April 3, 2023.

DOI: https://doi.org/10.2105/AJPH.2023.307311

CONFLICTS OF INTEREST

R. Hughes was vice president of public policy with Moderna during the COVID-19 pandemic.

REFERENCE

1. SteelFisher GK, Findling MG, Caporello HL, et al. Trust in US federal, state, and local public health agencies during COVID-19: responses and policy implications. *Health Aff (Millwood)*. 2023;42(3):328–337. https://doi.org/10.1377/hlthaff.2022.01204

Diversity of End-of-Life Care in the Boom of Deaths at Old Age

Qiushi Feng, PhD

ABOUT THE AUTHOR

Qiushi Feng is with the Department of Sociology and Anthropology and the Centre for Family and Population Research, National University of Singapore, Singapore.

See also Ebeling et al., p. 786.

The trend of prolonging life expectancy in the world population, though interrupted by the COVID-19 pandemic, is expected to resume soon, but whether the reduced mortality comes with less morbidity in later life is still debatable.[1] Despite such uncertainty, many aged societies in our world have started to see an unprecedented boom of deaths in their old-age populations. As highlighted by Ebeling et al. in the current issue of *AJPH* (p. 786), for example, Sweden will witness an annual increase of deaths by 25% in the next 30 years. By 2050, more than 30% of the world's countries are predicted to reach or surpass the current level of population aging in Sweden.[2] Thus, there has never been a better time to promote studies on death and dying among older people.

Ebeling et al. investigated changes in end-of-life care use among Swedish older people (≥ 70 years). It is comparable to an early study by Aaltonen et al.,[3] which examined the end-of-life care transfer of older people in Finland (≥ 70 years). Both studies utilized data on care use from the official registers of the respective countries and classified how end-of-life care is arranged at the population level. Based on data at two time points—two years and six months prior to death—the Finland study focused on care transfer between community, hospital, and residential care institution, reporting that about 60% of home dwellers moved to institutions or hospitals within the last six months of their lives. The current study on Sweden instead investigated a wide range of care use one year before death and at death, including home-based and institutional care as well as four medical services of clinical, acute, outpatient, and inpatient care. Six types of care use were identified: about 40% of people were categorized according to two "dependent" types (staying in a residential care institution and receiving either more or less medical care), whereas the other four types were all home dwellers, most receiving medical care. The current study, together with the Finland study and other related literature, revealed a great diversity of end-of-life care patterns, suggesting that the last stage of later life is uneven regarding where, when, and how various kinds of care are needed and delivered. This sends a strong message to stakeholders of the elder care sector, particularly given the escalating old-age deaths in many societies of the world.

Unlike in the Finland study, end-of-life transitions between home and a residential care institution were not common in Sweden as revealed by Ebeling et al. The use of medical services, however, was intensive in Sweden, although inpatient care was less utilized among older individuals living at home. One limitation of the current study, however, is the information shortage for the year prior to death. Taking into account the care situation at sixth months prior to death, which the literature shows is an important time-of-care changes in dying,[3,4] may help to capture more care transitions and yield a more valid typology. Moreover, the care classification in the current study was based on the Latent Class Analysis, a data-driven approach, so the conceptualization of these six types was based on summarized features of data clusters rather than direct empirical evidence. In this regard, there were efforts in the article to further examine the profiles of age, gender, and causes of death across the six groups, which enhanced the legitimacy of the classification. However, black boxes remain. For example, what kind of cancer was behind the group "terminal ill"? What type of cardiovascular disease was responsible for "sudden death"? And why were men more likely to be in the "terminal ill" group but women in the "dependent" group? Further work is called for to clarify mechanisms underlying the observed typology.

One essential point raised by Ebeling et al. is the contrast between the observed patterns of end-of-life care and the standard of a "good" death, which is expected to entail less care and more self-control. Such inconsistency is in line with the literature, which shows that a significant proportion of older people did not die at home even if they preferred to.[5] As implied by findings of the current study, the trend of

AJPH July 2023, Vol 113, No. 7

population aging is leading to more old-age deaths in residential care facilities. This may challenge the mainstream model of aging now in place and the ongoing movement toward deinstitutionalization.[6] With the mounting number of deaths with institutional long-term care, promoting aging-friendly residential care facilities with good end-of-life services becomes urgent. In this regard, as highlighted by Ebeling et al., how to help seniors afford such services is a valid concern, especially considering the present social inequality in dying.[7]

The multiple types of care use identified by the current study are considered by the authors to represent "fast and slowly progressing trajectories," the latter of which featured deaths in oldest old ages with a greater variation in causes of death. Consequently, the authors raised a meaningful hypothesis: the longer life span may partially come from a prolonged dying process with substantial care needs. This echoes well the classical hypothesis of morbidity expansion with population aging,[8] which predicts more morbidity with population aging among older people (failure) when life expectancy extends (success). In the ongoing debate between the failure of success versus success of success (or benefits of success vs costs of success),[9] the current study reminds us to give more weight to the end-of-life stage.

Lastly, the current study's applicability beyond Sweden is worth discussing, as the impact of increasing old-age deaths would differ by context. One recent article, for example, discussed the rise of old-age deaths in Japan, another world-leading nation in population aging.[10] Taking Japan as a "death-laden society," the author argued that the lack of end-of-life services, greater risk of lonely deaths, and debate on physician-assisted suicide could be eminent issues for Japan in the boom of old-age deaths.[10] In particular, given the specific socioeconomic and institutional context of the study by Ebeling et al., follow-up studies may pay attention to informal care by family members, which was not accounted for in the current study but is prevalent in non-Western societies.[11] AJPH

CORRESPONDENCE

Correspondence should be sent to Qiushi Feng, AS1 03-40, 11 Arts Link, Singapore 117570 (e-mail: socfq@nus.edu.sg). Reprints can be ordered at http://www.ajph.org by clicking the "Reprints" link.

PUBLICATION INFORMATION

Full Citation: Feng Q. Diversity of end-of-life care in the boom of deaths at old age. *Am J Public Health*. 2023;113(7):716–717.

Acceptance Date: April 12, 2023.

DOI: https://doi.org/10.2105/AJPH.2023.307319

CONFLICTS OF INTEREST

The author has no conflicts of interest to disclose.

REFERENCES

1. Robine JM, Jagger C, Crimmins EM, et al. Trends in health expectancies. In: Jagger C. Crimmins EM, Saito Y, et al., eds. *International Handbook of Health Expectancies.* Cham, Switzerland: Springer Nature; 2020:19–34. https://doi.org/10.1007/978-3-030-37668-0_2
2. Gu D, Andreev K, Dupre ME. Major trends in population growth around the world. *China CDC Wkly.* 2021;3(28):604–613. https://doi.org/10.46234/ccdcw2021.160
3. Aaltonen M, Forma L, Pulkki J, et al. Changes in older people's care profiles during the last 2 years of life, 1996–1998 and 2011–2013: a retrospective nationwide study in Finland. *BMJ Open.* 2017;7(11):e015130. https://doi.org/10.1136/bmjopen-2016-015130
4. Bähler C, Signorell A, Reich O. Health care utilisation and transitions between health care settings in the last 6 months of life in Switzerland. *PLoS One.* 2016;11(9):e0160932. https://doi.org/10.1371/journal.pone.0160932
5. Iyer AS, Brown CJ. End-of-life preferences in older US adults—bridging the "what matters" chasm. *JAMA Netw Open.* 2022;5(1):e2142279. https://doi.org/10.1001/jamanetworkopen.2021.42279
6. Anttonen A, Karsio O. Eldercare service redesign in Finland: deinstitutionalization of long-term care. *J Soc Serv Res.* 2016;42(2):151–166. https://doi.org/10.1080/01488376.2015.1129017
7. Hanratty B, Holmes L. Social inequality in dying. In: Oliviere D, Monroe B, Payne S, eds. *Death, Dying and Social Differences.* 2nd ed. Oxford, UK: Oxford University Press; 2011:19–31. https://doi.org/10.1093/acprof:oso/9780199599295.003.0014
8. Gruenberg EM. The failures of success. *Milbank Mem Fund Q Health Soc.* 1977;55(1):3–24. https://doi.org/10.2307/3349592
9. Zeng Y, Feng Q, Hesketh T, Christensen K, Vaupel JW. Survival, disabilities in activities of daily living, and physical and cognitive functioning among the oldest-old in China: a cohort study. *Lancet.* 2017;389(10079):1619–1629. https://doi.org/10.1016/S0140-6736(17)30548-2
10. Higo MA. "Death-laden society": the next stage of a hyper-aged Japan and health challenges ahead. *Aging Health Res.* 2022;2(4):100110. https://doi.org/10.1016/j.ahr.2022.100110
11. Feng Q, Straughan PT. What does successful aging mean? Lay perception of successful aging among Singapore elderly. *J Gerontol B Psychol Sci Soc Sci.* 2017;72(2):204–213. https://doi.org/10.1093/geronb/gbw151

To EHB 1638 or Not to EHB 1638? For Immunization Policymakers, That Is the Question

Joshua T. B. Williams, MD, and Sean T. O'Leary, MD, MPH

ABOUT THE AUTHORS

The authors are with the Department of Pediatrics, University of Colorado Anschutz Medical Campus, Aurora. Joshua T. B. Williams is with the Division of General Pediatrics, Ambulatory Care Services, Denver Health, Denver, CO. Sean T. O'Leary is also with the Division of Pediatric Infectious Diseases, Children's Hospital Colorado, Aurora.

See also Moore et al., p. 795.

Routine childhood immunizations are critical to our public health infrastructure. Vaccines protect individual children and indirectly protect others who cannot be immunized in their communities. An evaluation of the US immunization program for children in the 2017 birth cohort revealed that (1) routine immunization prevented more than 17 million cases of disease and 31 000 deaths, (2) 853 000 life-years and 892 000 quality-adjusted life-years were gained, and (3) estimated vaccination costs ($8.5 billion) were fully offset by the $63.6 billion in disease-related averted costs.[1]

These benefits have been recognized since the 19th century, when mandatory schooling and rising smallpox infection rates prompted the first policies requiring vaccination for school attendance. Children with medical contraindications were exempted, but from the outset policymakers struggled to balance legal compulsion and parental autonomy for those against vaccination. This struggle continued into the 20th century, when effective polio and measles vaccines were developed and states enacted myriad vaccination requirements.[2] Generally, laws required certain vaccines for school attendance, but they allowed exemptions for children on the grounds of religious or varied "personal" beliefs. States' laws continued to evolve in the second half of the 20th century as new vaccines were developed and legal challenges prompted exemption reforms to broadly accommodate a range of beliefs.[2]

Today all 50 states, the District of Columbia, and Puerto Rico have immunization requirements for child care centers and public schools.[3] Many private schools also have requirements. Although most children enter school or day care vaccinated, the rise of vaccine hesitancy and the disruption COVID-19 wrought on immunization delivery systems have caused multiyear declines in national vaccination coverage. During the 2021–2022 school year, coverage with two doses of measles, mumps, and rubella (MMR) vaccines among kindergartners fell to 93%, the lowest in a decade.[4] Nine states and the District of Columbia had coverage under 90%, or well below the estimated 95% threshold needed to prevent measles outbreaks.[4]

In this issue of *AJPH*, Moore et al. (p. 795) ask a simple question with important policy implications: what was the effect of Washington State's Engrossed House Bill (EHB) 1638, which removed personal belief exemptions for MMR vaccines only, on MMR completion and exemption rates among kindergarten through 12th-grade (K–12) students? EHB 1638 took effect in July 2019, and the authors looked backward to 2014 and forward to 2022 to estimate relative changes in kindergarten MMR vaccine completion rates and changes in exemption rates among K–12 students. In addition, the authors leveraged school- and county-level data to explore changes by school type (e.g., private vs public) and school district geographic areas. How did Washington's health policy experiment go?

According to the authors, it went well. EHB 1638 was associated with a 5.4% relative increase in kindergarten MMR completion rates and a 41% decrease in MMR exemptions for K–12 students; both findings were statistically significant. However, the rate of religious exemptions among all K–12 students for any required vaccine increased 367% after passage of the legislation; the rate of medical exemptions remained stable and was 0.7% in the 2021–2022 school year. Kindergartner MMR completion rate increases were not significantly different between public and private schools, but K–12 vaccine exemption rates rose significantly more in private schools. Results of spatial analyses showed that exemption rates declined in many school districts

AJPH July 2023, Vol 113, No. 7

with MMR exemption rates above 5% before the passage of EHB 1638 but that pre-passage exemption rates correlated highly with post-passage rates.

These findings are impressive. At first glance, one wants to agree with Moore et al. that "targeted policies that allow some NMEs [nonmedical exemptions] may be more effective than completely eliminating NMEs altogether." However, the authors stop short of recommending widespread implementation of policies akin to EHB 1638 across the United States, leaving public health and immunization advocates to debate "To EHB 1638 or not to EHB 1638?"

Proponents of targeted policies that eliminate nonmedical exemptions for selected vaccines will point to the apparent effectiveness of this bill at minimal cost. The 5% increase in kindergartner vaccination coverage, starting from a baseline rate of approximately 90%, is an important one. In communities with high coverage rates, incremental increases are usually achieved via exponentially costly interventions.[5] Yet, the gains after EHB 1638 were achieved through legislative action as opposed to a costly statewide immunization campaign. At a time of fiscal uncertainty, policymakers may especially appreciate and support immunization bills that improve public health without straining budgets.

Those in favor of targeted vaccination policies will also point to the stable proportion of children with medical exemptions during the postimplementation period. Previously, efforts to reform state immunization policies have caused rebound increases in medical exemptions that offset declines in nonmedical exemptions. For example, in 2016, California eliminated nonmedical exemptions. Shortly thereafter, clusters of medical exemptions appeared in areas that previously had high rates of nonmedical exemptions, and nearly 70% of the decreases in nonmedical exemptions initially observed were reversed.[6,7] The authors did not observe the same effect with the targeted approach of EHB 1638.

There are many concerns with EHB 1638, however. For instance, it led many vaccine-hesitant parents to use religious exemptions, creating a partial exemption replacement effect. We had previously observed this effect in the state of Vermont.[8] Although public health advocates will note that overall exemption rates still decreased, even with this replacement effect being taken into account, religious leaders may rightly object to the artificial creation of apparent religious resistance to vaccination across the state. Is it ethical to create apparent religious resistance to vaccines to decrease exemption rates? What say should faith leaders have? In 2019, after the measles outbreaks that prompted EHB 1638, the Archdiocese of Seattle—with more than 70 schools and 1 million members—stopped accepting religious vaccine exemptions in parochial schools.[9]

There are other important questions. If we develop targeted vaccination exemption policies, how do we decide on diseases and vaccines? EHB 1638 specified MMR, but most years many more children die from COVID-19, influenza, and pneumonia than contract measles in the United States, and thousands of adults die from vaccine-preventable diseases related to human papillomavirus.[10] As others have noted, eliminating nonmedical exemptions for MMR only could lead parents to the misperception that MMR is the only vaccine truly needed for child health and that others are simply a matter of personal preference.[11] Do we dare venture down this slippery slope?

Another question: should we model policies after one that is inequitable? With EHB 1638, parents of children in private schools—who, presumably, have more resources and flexibility than parents of children in public schools—found physicians willing to provide their children with medical exemptions or filed the appropriate paperwork for religious exemptions. Finally, how certain are we that the effects of EHB 1638 will continue? In the study's final year, the COVID-19 public health emergency was ongoing. Will replacement effects grow as monitoring continues? Correctly, the authors note that more observation is needed.

Ultimately, for policy experts seeking direction, EHB 1638 poses more questions than it answers. For these reasons and many others, all major professional societies, including the American Public Health Association and the American Academy of Pediatrics, advocate for the complete elimination of nonmedical vaccine exemptions.[12] Nevertheless, this is a welcome addition to the vaccine exemption literature, and it suggests that EHB 1638 has, for a time, improved the safety of children and communities throughout Washington. AJPH

CORRESPONDENCE

Correspondence should be sent to Joshua T. B. Williams, MD, 301 W 6th Ave, MC 1911, Denver, CO 80204 (e-mail: joshua.williams@dhha.org). Reprints can be ordered at http://www.ajph.org by clicking the "Reprints" link.

PUBLICATION INFORMATION

Full Citation: Williams JTB, O'Leary ST. To EHB 1638 or not to EHB 1638? for immunization policymakers, that is the question. *Am J Public Health*. 2023;113(7):718–720.

Acceptance Date: April 12, 2023.

DOI: https://doi.org/10.2105/AJPH.2023.307318

CONTRIBUTORS

J. T. B. Williams conceptualized, drafted, and revised the editorial. S. T. O'Leary critically reviewed and revised the editorial.

CONFLICTS OF INTEREST

The authors report no potential or actual conflicts of interest from funding or affiliation-related activities pertinent to this editorial.

REFERENCES

1. Carrico J, La EM, Talbird SE, et al. Value of the Immunization Program for Children in the 2017 US birth cohort. *Pediatrics.* 2022;150(3):e2021056007. https://doi.org/10.1542/peds.2021-056007
2. Conis E. The history of the personal belief exemption. *Pediatrics.* 2020;145(4):e20192551. https://doi.org/10.1542/peds.2019-2551
3. National Conference of State Legislatures. States with religious and philosophical exemptions to school immunization requirements. Available at: https://www.ncsl.org/health/states-with-religious-and-philosophical-exemptions-from-school-immunization-requirements. Accessed April 3, 2023.
4. Seither R, Calhoun K, Yusuf OB, et al. Vaccination coverage with selected vaccines and exemption rates among children in kindergarten—United States, 2021–22 school year. *MMWR Morb Mortal Wkly Rep.* 2023;72(2):26–32. https://doi.org/10.15585/mmwr.mm7202a2
5. Ozawa S, Yemeke TT, Thompson KM. Systematic review of the incremental costs of interventions that increase immunization coverage. *Vaccine.* 2018;36(25):3641–3649. https://doi.org/10.1016/j.vaccine.2018.05.030
6. Delamater PL, Leslie TF, Yang YT. Change in medical exemptions from immunization in California after elimination of personal belief exemptions. *JAMA.* 2017;318(9):863–864. https://doi.org/10.1001/jama.2017.9242
7. Delamater PL, Pingali SC, Buttenheim AM, Salmon DA, Klein NP, Omer SB. Elimination of nonmedical immunization exemptions in California and school-entry vaccine status. *Pediatrics.* 2019;143(6):e20183301. https://doi.org/10.1542/peds.2018-3301
8. Williams JTB, Rice J, Cox-Martin M, Bayliss EA, O'Leary ST. Religious vaccine exemptions in kindergartners: 2011–2018. *Pediatrics.* 2019;144(6):e20192710. https://doi.org/10.1542/peds.2019-2710
9. Northwest Catholic. School immunization policy updated to reflect Catholic teaching. Available at: https://www.nwcatholic.org/news/local/school-immunization-policy-updated-to-reflect-catholic-teaching.html. Accessed August 12, 2020.
10. National Center for Health Statistics. Pneumonia and influenza mortality surveillance. Available at: https://gis.cdc.gov/grasp/fluview/mortality.html. Accessed April 3, 2023.
11. Byington CL, Clayton EW, Edwards KM. Childhood vaccine exemptions: a broader perspective is required. *Pediatrics.* 2016;137(4):e20160189. https://doi.org/10.1542/peds.2016-0189
12. American Academy of Pediatrics. Medical versus nonmedical immunization exemptions for child care and school attendance. *Pediatrics.* 2016;138(3):e20162145. https://doi.org/10.1542/peds.2016-2145

Probability Samples Provide a Means of Benchmarking and Adjusting for Data Collected From Nonprobability Samples

Michael R. Elliott, PhD

ABOUT THE AUTHOR

Michael R. Elliott is with the University of Michigan School of Public Health, Biostatics, and the Institute for Social Research, Survey Methodology Program, Ann Arbor.

See also Keith et al., p. 768.

I want to thank Keith et al. (p. 768) for an important exploration of the much-neglected problem of obtaining accurate estimates of the COVID-19 pandemic spread in real time. The authors compared a standard probability sample with a convenience sample (each with about a 1% finite population fraction) and administrative records to estimate seroprevalence of COVID-19 in Jefferson County, Kentucky. Jefferson County is essentially Louisville and the immediate suburbs, with a population of approximately 800 000.[1] They found little difference between the probability sample and the convenience sample with respect to either the distribution of covariates or the prevalence estimates after raking both samples to known sex, race, and geographic region, but substantial differences between the prevalence estimates from the sampling methods and the administrative record estimates.

The results provide important findings that in some ways match prior expectations and in other ways defy them. First, the sample-based estimates of prevalence are higher than prevalences obtained from the administrative records, and the authors assume that sample-based estimates are more accurate. The authors do not state exactly why they make this assumption, but it is presumably because administrative records require a reported positive test filed with Louisville Metro Public Health and Wellness and thus exclude nearly all cases that were asymptomatic, as well as cases that did not result in a visit to a physician or testing site. Assuming that the sample estimates are the "gold standard," this leads to an underreporting by two factors or more, and perhaps even higher among minorities. This is not a novel finding,[2,3] but it confirms some previous literature in the area and provides a rough estimate of the magnitude by which administratively reported cases (which constitute the vast bulk of prevalence data in both the United States and around the world) should be multiplied to obtain an estimate of the true number of cases, at least during the 2020–2021 period.

The second finding—that the probability sample and the convenience sample prevalence estimates correspond—contradicts a nontrivial body of literature that suggests that even low-response-rate probability samples can yield more accurate results than convenience samples. Kennedy et al.[4] found major quality concerns using on-line panel convenience samples with respect to the measurement of US political attitudes and recreational interests, especially for Black and Hispanic samples, although there was substantial variation in quality among vendors. In a major study that compared both random digit-dial (RDD) and address-based sampling-web (ABS-web) probability samples with six nonprobability samples with respect to a variety of demographic, health, economic, and transportation measures, MacInnis et al.[5] found that the probability samples performed substantially better when benchmarked against high-quality census data obtained by the Current Population Survey, the Current Expenditure Survey, or National Center for Health Statistics surveys such as the National Health Interview Survey or the National Health and Nutrition Examination Survey. Furthermore, Groves and Peytcheva[6] found that nonresponse rates were only weakly linked to nonresponse bias in a large meta-analysis. Further work by Tourangeau[7] and by Brick and Tourangeau[8] explained this finding by arguing that most nonresponse is due to missing completely at random[9] factors (i.e., factors completely independent of any data being collected from participants) such as happenstance of contact time or study-level design features unrelated to sampled member characteristics, or to participant-level characteristics unrelated to survey variables. Thus, it is somewhat surprising that even a low-response-rate survey did not differ to some degree from a volunteer sample. Although the authors cite 30% as a "safe" cutoff for response rates,[10] MacInnis and colleagues' RDD and ABS-web probability samples had response rates of 15% and 2%, respectively, yet still dominated their convenience sample competitors with respect to bias. It may be that, with their response rates of 2% to 5% (depending on region of the county), Keith et al. have finally descended into volunteer territory, especially given that the data collection required the respondent to make an in-person visit to a separate clinic.

As a survey statistician, I became enormously frustrated that nearly a century of learning how to obtain accurate prevalence estimates from a population appeared to be all but forgotten in this public health crisis. Systems such as the Behavioral Risk Factor Surveillance System that had been put into place long ago to provide flexible, real-time data collection on "emerging public health problems"[11] were not up to the task, given the speed of infectious disease spread. As noted by Keith et al., there have been a few attempts to use traditional methods. For example, in a study somewhat similar to that of the authors, Menachemi et al.[12] conducted a study in Indiana with 68 statewide testing facilities, obtaining a considerably higher 24% response rate. Their resulting estimate of population prevalence early in the pandemic (2.8% at the end of April 2020) was far higher than the rate obtained from the number of confirmed cases at the Indiana State Department of Health (0.3% of the population); despite the higher response rate, racial minorities were severely undersampled (8% non-White vs 23% in the population, and 2% Hispanic vs 8% in the population; estimates were postratified to age, gender, and race distributions). Although there are no "gold standards" to assess prevalence measures, the resulting derived case-fatality rate was 0.58% at the time, consistent with the 0.66% Chinese fatality rate estimated at that time after careful adjustment for censoring and ascertainment bias.[13] On the other hand, major nonprobability samples such as Delphi-Facebook[14] were shown to perform poorly when estimating COVID-19 vaccine uptake compared with the probability sample obtained from Ipsos online KnowledgePanel,[15] even though the latter had only a 10.5% response rate.[16] Although hardly a complete literature review of a still evolving "autopsy" of the failure of the public health and medical community to grapple with this aspect of the COVID-19 pandemic response, it does suggest that a more nimble and survey science–informed response may have been helpful. Survey researchers could have perhaps been more creative in suggesting alternatives to standard methods (e.g., use of at-door drop boxes rather than requiring travel to remote sites), although undoubtedly many such suggestions would have foundered on blanket data collection shutdowns of survey-related research.

In sum, although Keith et al. provide an example in which probability sampling and convenience sampling gave similar results, I believe a broader overview still suggests the need for probability samples to provide a means of benchmarking and adjusting for data collected from nonprobability samples.[17,18] For an excellent example of this approach applied to prevalence estimates that leverage the previously mentioned Indiana study in combination with an Indianapolis-only probability sample, state-level Delphi-Facebook reports of symptoms, and administrative COVID-19 death data, see Dempsey.[19] Dempsey develops a procedure that combines administrative case-count data, data from nonprobability samples, and data from random samples over time to estimate selection propensities based on key covariate information. These selection propensities are then combined with epidemiological forecast models to construct a doubly robust estimator that accounts for both measurement-error and selection bias to estimate population seropositivity. AJPH

CORRESPONDENCE

Correspondence should be sent to Michael R. Elliott, M4124 SPHII, 1415 Washington Heights, Ann Arbor, MI 48109 (e-mail: mrelliot@umich.edu). Reprints can be ordered at http://www.ajph.org by clicking the "Reprints" link.

PUBLICATION INFORMATION

Full Citation: Elliott MR. Probability samples provide a means of benchmarking and adjusting for data collected from nonprobability samples. *Am J Public Health*. 2023;113(7):721–723.

Acceptance Date: April 12, 2023.

DOI: https://doi.org/10.2105/AJPH.2023.307317

CONFLICTS OF INTEREST

The author has no conflicts of interest to disclose.

REFERENCES

1. US Census Bureau. QuickFacts: Jefferson County, Kentucky. Available at: https://www.census.gov/quickfacts/jeffersoncountykentucky. Accessed April 9, 2023.
2. Albani V, Loria J, Massad E, Zubelli J. COVID-19 underreporting and its impact on vaccination strategies. *BMC Infect Dis.* 2021;21(1):1111. https://doi.org/10.1186/s12879-021-06780-7
3. Schwab N, Nienhold R, Henkel M, et al. COVID-19 autopsies reveal underreporting of SARS-CoV-2 infection and scarcity of co-infections. *Front Med (Lausanne).* 2022;9: 868954. https://doi.org/10.3389/fmed.2022.868954
4. Kennedy C, Mercer A, Keeter S, et al. *Evaluating Online Nonprobability Surveys.* Washington, DC: Pew Research Center; 2016:61.
5. MacInnis B, Krosnick JA, Ho AS, Cho MJ. The accuracy of measurements with probability and nonprobability survey samples: replication and extension.

Public Opin Q. 2018;82(4):707–744. https://doi.org/10.1093/poq/nfy038

6. Groves RM, Peytcheva E. The impact of nonresponse rates on nonresponse bias: a meta-analysis. *Public Opin Q.* 2008;72(2):167–189. https://doi.org/10.1093/poq/nfn011
7. Tourangeau R. Presidential address: paradoxes of nonresponse. *Public Opin Q.* 2017;81(3):803–814. https://doi.org/10.1093/poq/nfx031
8. Brick J, Tourangeau R. Responsive survey designs for reducing nonresponse bias. *J Off Stat.* 2017; 33(3):735–752. https://doi.org/10.1515/jos-2017-0034
9. Little RJA, Rubin DB. *Statistical Analysis With Missing Data.* 3rd ed. Hoboken, NJ: John Wiley & Sons; 2020.
10. Hedlin D. Is there a "safe area" where the nonresponse rate has only a modest effect on bias despite non-ignorable nonresponse? *Int Stat Rev.* 2020;88(3):642–657. https://doi.org/10.1111/insr.12359
11. Remington PL, Smith MY, Williamson DF, et al. Design, characteristics, and usefulness of state-based behavioral risk factor surveillance: 1981–87. *Public Health Rep.* 1988;103(4):366–375.
12. Menachemi N, Yiannoutsos CT, Dixon BE, et al. Population point prevalence of SARS-CoV-2 infection based on a statewide random sample—Indiana, April 25–29, 2020. *MMWR Morb Mortal Wkly Rep.* 2020;69(29):960–964. https://doi.org/10.15585/mmwr.mm6929e1
13. Verity R, Okell LC, Dorigatti I, et al. Estimates of the severity of coronavirus disease 2019: a model-based analysis. *Lancet Infect Dis.* 2020;20(6): 669–677. https://doi.org/10.1016/S1473-3099(20)30243-7
14. Salomon JA, Reinhart A, Bilinski A, et al. The US COVID-19 Trends and Impact Survey: continuous real-time measurement of COVID-19 symptoms, risks, protective behaviors, testing, and vaccination. *Proc Natl Acad Sci U S A.* 2021;118(51): e2111454118. https://doi.org/10.1073/pnas.2111454118
15. Bradley VC, Kuriwaki S, Isakov M, et al. Unrepresentative big surveys significantly overestimated US vaccine uptake. *Nature.* 2021;600(7890): 695–700. https://doi.org/10.1038/s41586-021-04198-4
16. Consumer and Community Research Section of the Federal Reserve Board's Division of Consumer and Community Affairs. Economic Well-Being of US Households in 2020–May 2021. Available at: https://www.federalreserve.gov/publications/2021-economic-well-being-of-us-households-in-2020-acknowledgments.htm. Accessed April 9, 2023.
17. Elliott MR, Valliant R. Inference for nonprobability samples. *Stat Sci.* 2017;32(2):249–264. https://doi.org/10.1214/16-STS598
18. Wu C. Statistical inference with non-probability survey samples. *Surv Methodol.* 2022;48(2): 283–311.
19. Dempsey W. Addressing selection bias and measurement error in COVID-19 case count data using auxiliary information. *Ann Appl Stat.* In press.

It's the Smoke, Not the Fire

David P. Eisenman, MD, MSHS

ABOUT THE AUTHOR

David P. Eisenman is professor of medicine at the David Geffen School of Medicine, director of the Center for Public Health and Disasters, and codirector of the Center for Healthy Climate Solutions, School of Public Health, University of California, Los Angeles.

See also Vargo et al., p. 759.

Most Americans are breathing increasingly unhealthy air from wildfire smoke. This is the first conclusion of the study by Vargo et al. in this issue of *AJPH* (p. 759) quantifying the magnitude of a growing climate change hazard in the United States, namely exposure to the toxic smoke of wildland fires. These increases are happening across both advantaged and disadvantaged communities. This is the second, and more important, conclusion because it counters the dominant media narrative that wildfires are an affliction of the rich. This study highlights the need for public health to do more to protect socially disadvantaged groups and to direct national attention to the smoke and away from the flames.

Climate change is producing longer fire seasons, with more frequent and severe wildfires. The resulting smoke is a complex mixture of corrosive gases and carcinogenic compounds, including particulate matter less than 2.5 microns in diameter ($PM_{2.5}$)—a toxic mixture of solid and liquid particles that gets into the bloodstream. $PM_{2.5}$ causes a wide range of physical, mental, developmental, and cognitive health harms.

The smoke can travel thousands of kilometers from its source, polluting distant communities for weeks and months. For instance, forest fires in Quebec, Canada, led to air pollution in Baltimore, Maryland, with peak $PM_{2.5}$ values 17 times higher than the Environmental Protection Agency's National Ambient Air Quality standards and to increased cardiorespiratory hospitalization rates across the mid-Atlantic and Northeastern United States.[1,2] Although large fires more often occur in the Western United States, much of the attributable mortality and morbidity may occur in the Eastern United States because of its higher population density.[3] As the world enters a time of increasing wildfires, chronic, multiweek fires—as were seen in Australia in 2019 and California in 2020—will become more usual.

With this background in mind, consider the study by Vargo et al. of national-level trends in smoke exposure from 2011 to 2021 and their intersections with social vulnerability.

The authors combined satellite data on wildfire smoke plumes with US Census population data. They assigned daily smoke plume densities (high, medium, light, none) to each census block group and its 2010 population. Person-days of smoke, which is the product of the number of people in a census block group and the number of days that block group experienced smoke, were summed to the census tract to estimate exposure levels.

The results are alarming. Across the United States we are exposed to more wildfire smoke, and few counties are unaffected. The five-year annual average exposure to heavy smoke increased 350%, from 307 million person-days during 2011 to 2015 to 1.381 billion person-days during 2017 to 2021. The authors estimate a total of 2.9 billion person-days of heavy smoke across the US population in 2021 (the US population was 331.9 million people in 2021). More than 87% of the US population experienced increases in the number of days of heavy smoke between these periods. Light smoke days increased too, which is important because there is likely no "safe" level[4] of exposure to pollutants such as $PM_{2.5}$. Eastern states experienced these increases too, albeit starting from a lower baseline. Wildfire smoke has become everyone's problem.

Protecting oneself from wildfire smoke is difficult when it requires staying indoors in homes with air conditioners and good air filtration, avoiding outdoor work, avoiding traveling (so working from home), and even temporarily leaving your home to stay in places beyond the spreading smoke. As in disasters generally, the level of population harm is a product of social disadvantage and the capacity to protect oneself from the hazard. For instance, infiltration of outdoor pollutants into homes is higher on average for older, smaller homes and for lower-income households, and these differences could lead to disparities in overall individual exposure even if ambient exposures are equivalent.[5] This is where the second part of the authors' results fits in.

The authors used the Centers for Disease Control and Prevention's Social Vulnerability Index to investigate characteristics that might affect the health

AJPH July 2023, Vol 113, No. 7

risks of smoke exposure. This index contains census-derived data on sociodemographic, economic, and cultural characteristics, which the authors used to rank census tracts by their levels of social disadvantage. Census tracts at the greatest social disadvantage experienced a 358% increase in the average annual number of heavy smoke days, from 0.92 days in 2011 to 2015 to 4.21 days in 2017 to 2021.

Census tracts with relative advantage showed similar, if not higher, increases in heavy smoke person-days (annual number of heavy smoke days of 1.13 in 2011–2015 to 4.79 days in 2017–2021). Still, this study highlights inequities of the utmost importance. Although everyone is seeing more exposure, those with the greatest disadvantage often start from a baseline of worse health, have the least access to protections, and have more frequent health harms. Add wildfire smoke to the list of inequities that climate change is worsening.

Vargo et al. note that their results may represent the upper bound of estimates because they used satellite plume data rather than ground-level measurements of air quality—the smoke could be aloft and captured by satellites but not be affecting the ground where people are breathing. Still, even more conservative estimates demand our attention and response.[6] Because disadvantaged communities are more prone to suffer from disaster impacts, any meaningful discussion of wildfire smoke needs to address this health equity issue.

The media's penchant for photographing large homes burning in Western mountains depicts wildfires as a problem mainly for wealthy owners of second homes in California and the West. But it is the smoke, not the fire. We in public health must redirect media attention to the problem as we know it really is experienced—households near and far from the fire are suffering harms, hospitalizations, and deaths from the smoke menacing our air.

Additional quantitative and qualitative investigation is necessary to gain a deeper understanding of the relationship between social vulnerability and the health effects of smoke. Studies like that of Vargo et al. analyze vulnerability factors independently when it is likely they are operating synergistically. We need better measures of indoor exposure, as the most common advisory during an event is to stay indoors, but poor housing quality may reduce the benefits. We also need to analyze social vulnerability at smaller scales to better understand local impacts, for instance, combining fine-resolution geospatial data with the rich data available in electronic medical record systems to identify subpopulations most harmed by wildfire smoke.

Focusing our public health interventions on the communities with social disadvantages may maximize our impact, and we need program evaluations to assess this. The accelerating increase in smoke exposure calls for new approaches too. For instance, public health recommendations for protection from wildfire smoke include staying indoors in homes equipped with an air purifier and a HEPA (high-efficiency particulate air) filter. As the authors point out, this is a costly protection beyond the reach of many households. Publicly financed housing modifications, such as retrofits and air purification, may be required in communities with high exposures and high social vulnerability.

During the 2020 California wildfires, the Bay Area Air Quality Management District provided portable air filtration units to low-income individuals on Medi-Cal with severe asthma or other respiratory conditions. More public health departments should identify socially disadvantaged neighborhoods and prioritize those that need increased wildfire smoke preparedness messages, supplies, and access to clean air shelters.

The point is the smoke. AJPH

CORRESPONDENCE

Correspondence should be sent to David P. Eisenman, Division of General Internal Medicine and Health Services Research, 1100 Glendon Ave, Suite 850-878, Los Angeles, CA 90024 (e-mail: deisenman@mednet.ucla.edu). Reprints can be ordered at http://www.ajph.org by clicking the "Reprints" link.

PUBLICATION INFORMATION

Full Citation: Eisenman DP. It's the smoke, not the fire. *Am J Public Health*. 2023;113(7):724–725.

Acceptance Date: April 21, 2023.

DOI: https://doi.org/10.2105/AJPH.2023.307327

CONFLICTS OF INTEREST

The author has no conflicts of interest to declare.

REFERENCES

1. Sapkota A, Symons JM, Kleissl J, et al. Impact of the 2002 Canadian forest fires on particulate matter air quality in Baltimore City. *Environ Sci Technol*. 2005;39(1):24–32. https://doi.org/10.1021/es035311z
2. Le GE, Breysse P, McDermott A, et al. Canadian forest fires and the effects of long-range transboundary air pollution on hospitalizations among the elderly. *ISPRS Int J Geoinf*. 2014;3(2):713–731. https://doi.org/10.3390/ijgi3020713
3. O'Dell K, Bilsback K, Ford B, et al. Estimated mortality and morbidity attributable to smoke plumes in the United States: not just a Western US problem. *Geohealth*. 2021;5(9):e2021GH000457. https://doi.org/10.1029/2021GH000457
4. Di Q, Wang Y, Zanobetti A, et al. Air pollution and mortality in the Medicare population. *N Engl J Med*. 2017;376(26):2513–2522. https://doi.org/10.1056/NEJMoa1702747
5. Chan WR, Joh J, Sherman MH. Analysis of air leakage measurements of US houses. *Energy Build*. 2013;66:616–625. https://doi.org/10.1016/j.enbuild.2013.07.047
6. Childs ML, Li J, Wen J, et al. Daily local-level estimates of ambient wildfire smoke $PM_{2.5}$ for the contiguous US. *Environ Sci Technol*. 2022;56(19):13607–13621. https://doi.org/10.1021/acs.est.2c02934

Mortality Inequities: Power, Theory, and Data Considerations

Jaquelyn L. Jahn, PhD, MPH, and Stephanie M. Hernandez, PhD, MS

ABOUT THE AUTHORS

Both authors are with the Drexel University Dornsife School of Public Health, Philadelphia, PA.

Some of the earliest epidemiological work identified mortality gaps across social class, with differing theoretical approaches as to how these inequities should be measured, interpreted, and intervened in.[1] Today, most social epidemiological research takes a "gradational" approach, demonstrating greater risk of mortality across continuous indicators, such as income, wealth, and educational attainment.[2] In the June issue of *AJPH*, Eisenberg-Guyot et al. (https://bit.ly/3oEmOu0) break from the gradational tradition by applying a Marxist understanding of social class in their examination of mortality across business owners (incorporated and unincorporated), managers, workers, and those not in the labor force—categories they constructed to indicate power over productive property and workers' labor.

The article's novel operationalization results from a relational understanding of social class, that is, that class positions reflect how power is inequitably held and the oppressive means through which it is maintained. Although a gradational approach has certainly produced population health research that is informative for social policy, showing the health impacts of compulsory schooling or the Earned Income Tax Credit for example,[2] a relational approach, like the one Eisenberg-Guyot et al. demonstrate, challenges public health researchers and practitioners to question how power operates through broader economic and political systems, how these systems produce health inequities, and how they might be changed. We use the incisive article of Eisenberg-Guyot et al. as an example to structure a discussion on why bringing an analysis of power relations is important for health equity and how public health research can illustrate how capitalism operates alongside other systems of oppression. We also describe theories and frameworks that can support this work and related challenges and opportunities in population health data collection.

POWER RELATIONS

An analysis of power relations is missing from the theories that guide mainstream epidemiological research.[1] The article by Eisenberg-Guyot et al. illustrates what is made possible by this kind of shift in thinking about social stratification and, particularly, why it matters for the measurement and interpretation of health inequities. Through their operationalization of social class, Eisenberg-Guyot et al. expand the focus beyond solely identifying the health harms of poverty, income, or other socioeconomic determinants of health and instead explore which groups profit and whose health is protected at the expense of others. This theoretical orientation moves population health research toward asking questions about how health inequities arise from patterns of consumption, resource extraction, privatization, profiteering, and opportunity hoarding, for example.

Relational thinking can be guided by some theories of disease distribution, including the political economy of health and ecosocial theory,[1] and there are also several frameworks from disciplines outside public health that can support this kind of research. For instance, intersectionality emphasizes that identities (e.g., one's class, race, or gender) matter as attributes of individuals but more importantly because they reflect differences in power that interact with and reinforce systems of privilege and oppression.[3,4] The specificity that intersectionality demands is critical because, as Crenshaw explained:

> Where systems of race, gender, and class domination converge, intervention strategies based solely on the experiences of women [or people of any gender] who do not share the same class or race backgrounds will be of limited help to women [or people of that same gender] who face different obstacles because of race and class.[5(p1246)]

Importantly, Eisenberg-Guyot et al. bring to their class analysis a discussion of structural racism and sexism as coproducing social class inequities in mortality. They find that 25% of non-Hispanic White men were business owners or managers versus 10% of Black women and that there are greater class inequities in mortality among minoritized racial and ethnic groups

AJPH July 2023, Vol 113, No. 7

than among White respondents. The authors underscore that structural racism and sexism drive certain groups into exploitative and more dangerous working conditions as well as (and because of) concentrated class power among employers.

Recent articles have also called attention to racial capitalism's role in disease distribution and etiology, particularly using the example of inequities in COVID-19 mortality.[6–8] Ruth Wilson Gilmore describes inequities in mortality as part of the very definition of racism: "the state-sanctioned or extralegal production and exploitation of group-differentiated vulnerability to premature death."[9(p28)] Embedded in this definition is an understanding of racism and capitalism as mutually reinforcing: the exploitation of racially minoritized groups is part of how capitalism works, which in turn is part of racialization. In this view, it is futile to attempt to separate the effects of race and class on health inequities, and, moreover, thinking about capitalism is integral to understanding structural racism.

Eisenberg-Guyot et al. hypothesize that occupational hazards and exploitative working conditions likely contributed to the sharply differentiated survival curves shown across race and class. The lowest survival rates, by far, were observed among working-age adults who were not in the labor force. Thinking about power relations under racial capitalism can inform analyses of who might be included in this category, considering, for example, how certain groups—sexual and gender minorities and especially transgender people, Black or Indigenous people and other people of color, undocumented people—are disproportionately criminalized, incarcerated, and consequently removed from or marginalized in the labor market (although, currently, incarcerated people are excluded from the data used in this study, a limitation that we elaborate on in the "Data Challenges" section).

Applying a clear analysis of power relations matters not only for constructing and interpreting health inequities across social categories; relational thinking also brings forth a different set of strategies to reduce health inequities.[1] Eisenberg-Guyot et al. call for interventions that would build collective power among workers and other marginalized groups, such as unionization and decommodification, guaranteeing access to basic life necessities such as utilities, stable housing, and universal health care. This theoretical perspective is especially relevant in a political moment of egregiously high rates of COVID-19 mortality among low-wage "essential workers" and racially minoritized populations globally, alongside the sunsetting of pandemic welfare policies in the United States.[6] We caution, however, that public health researchers and practitioners must simultaneously recognize how social protections and power-building efforts are and are not designed to serve all marginalized groups (e.g., domestic workers, undocumented people). After all, no research or practice can truly be intersectional without a commitment to the advancement of social justice.

DATA CHALLENGES

The relational social class measure that Eisenberg-Guyot et al. developed invites a conversation on the measurement of social class in population surveys and, more broadly, the need for public health data that reflect relational thinking. Although the National Health Interview Survey (NHIS) used in this analysis does measure business ownership, occupation, and employment status, the lack of consistent data on supervisor status, for example, illustrates the larger problem of population surveys not being set up for this type of inquiry.

Similarly, the authors discuss limitations in how gender was classified using a binary male–female sex variable assigned by study interviewers, potentially misclassifying transgender and nonbinary respondents. The inability to identify transgender individuals and other gender minorities has meaningful implications for understanding occupational segregation and labor force participation. Estimates from the 2015 United States Transgender Survey suggest that, among respondents who held a job in the past year, nearly one in three (30%) reported some form of mistreatment (e.g., getting fired or being denied a promotion) related to their gender identity or expression.[10] It is important to note that although NHIS has been collected since 1957, as of 2023, there are no measures of gender identity or gender expression in the NHIS, and it took more than 50 years for a question on sexual orientation to be added. These three dimensions of social stratification have substantial implications for occupational segregation and the related risk of premature death.

In addition to measurement, Eisenberg-Guyot et al. identified challenges with sampling, particularly in that they needed to aggregate respondents into one racially minoritized group because of small cell sizes. Had the authors been able to disaggregate by race and gender in addition to social class, or had they been able to include currently incarcerated and other institutionalized populations excluded from the NHIS, wider inequities would likely have been observed. To address the underrepresentation of certain marginalized groups in population surveys, sampling strategies will need to be changed[11] while being cognizant of respondent burden, decreasing response rates in federal surveys, and ensuring respondent confidentiality. Intersectionality can help guide these data collection efforts.[4]

CONCLUSIONS

The article by Eisenberg-Guyot et al. starkly contrasts the realities of living and dying across social class strata in the United States and, in doing so, amplifies the need to change the structures that produce these inequities. Their relational operationalization of social class is a significant contribution to public health research, and it should also be acknowledged that their work echoes what social movements have already been articulating. Movement builders have long worked toward shifting power relations while also contributing to social theory on these issues. Claudia Jones (1915–1964), for example, was a Black woman, anti-imperialist, antifascist, leading theoretician in the Communist Party USA. Her writing on the "super-exploitation" of Black women identifies the gendered racism experienced by Black working-class women, and she did so for the express purpose of political mobilization.[12] Similarly, the Combahee River Collective contributed theory that is foundational to intersectionality's structural understanding of identity, while simultaneously building collective identity as a political project.[3] Our hope is not only that the relational theorizing demonstrated by Eisenberg-Guyot et al. sparks greater researcher recognition for the centrality of capitalism and power relations in producing health inequities but also that we do so to further our collective liberation in the real world. AJPH

CORRESPONDENCE

Correspondence should be sent to Jaquelyn L. Jahn, 3600 Market St, Room 727, Philadelphia, PA 19104 (e-mail: jackie.jahn@drexel.edu). Reprints can be ordered at http://www.ajph.org by clicking the "Reprints" link.

PUBLICATION INFORMATION

Full Citation: Jahn JL, Hernandez SM. Mortality inequities: power, theory, and data considerations. *Am J Public Health*. 2023;113(7):726–728.

Acceptance Date: April 15, 2023.

DOI: https://doi.org/10.2105/AJPH.2023.307322

CONTRIBUTORS

The authors both contributed to writing and editing the editorial.

ACKNOWLEDGMENTS

We would like to thank Gabe Schwartz for feedback on an early draft of the editorial.

CONFLICTS OF INTEREST

The authors have no conflicts of interest to declare.

REFERENCES

1. Krieger N. *Epidemiology and the People's Health: Theory and Context*. Oxford Academic online edition; May 1, 2011. Available at: https://doi.org/10.1093/acprof:oso/9780195383874.001.0001. Accessed April 19, 2023.
2. Glymour MM, Avendano M, Kawachi I. Socioeconomic status and health. In: Berkman LF, Kawachi I, Glymour MM, eds. *Social Epidemiology*. 2nd ed. New York, NY: Oxford University Press; 2014: 17–62. https://doi.org/10.1093/med/9780195377903.003.0002
3. Hill Collins P, Bilge S. *Intersectionality*. Cambridge, UK: Polity Press; 2016.
4. Bowleg L. Evolving intersectionality within public health: from analysis to action. *Am J Public Health*. 2021;111(1):88–90. https://doi.org/10.2105/AJPH.2020.306031
5. Crenshaw K. Mapping the margins: intersectionality, identity politics, and violence against women of color. *Stanford Law Rev*. 1991;43(6):1241–1299. https://doi.org/10.2307/1229039
6. Taiwo OO, Fehrenbacher AE, Cooke A. Material insecurity, racial capitalism, and public health. *Hastings Cent Rep*. 2021;51(6):17–22. https://doi.org/10.1002/hast.1293
7. Laster Pirtle WN. Racial capitalism: a fundamental cause of novel coronavirus (COVID-19) pandemic inequities in the United States. *Health Educ Behav*. 2020;47(4):504–508. https://doi.org/10.1177/1090198120922942
8. McClure ES, Vasudevan P, Bailey Z, Patel S, Robinson WR. Racial capitalism within public health—how occupational settings drive COVID-19 disparities. *Am J Epidemiol*. 2020;189(11):1244–1253. https://doi.org/10.1093/aje/kwaa126
9. Wilson Gilmore R, *Golden Gulag: Prisons, Surplus, and Opposition in Globalizing California*. Berkeley, CA: University of California Press; 2007.
10. James SE, Herman JL, Rankin S, Keisling M, Mottet L, Anafi M. *The Report of the 2015 US Transgender Survey*. Washington, DC: National Center for Transgender Equality; 2016. Available at: https://transequality.org/sites/default/files/docs/usts/USTS-Full-Report-Dec17.pdf. Accessed April 19, 2023.
11. Hernandez SM, Sparks PJ. Barriers to health care among adults with minoritized identities in the United States, 2013–2017. *Am J Public Health*. 2020;110(6):857–862. https://doi.org/10.2105/AJPH.2020.305598
12. Carole BD. *Left of Karl Marx: The Political Life of Black Communist Claudia Jones*. Durham, NC: Duke University Press; 2008.

An Equity-Focused Care Continuum Framework for Mpox and Future Infectious Disease Outbreaks: A Public Health of Consequence, July 2023

Robert A. Pitts, MD, Angelica Cifuentes Kottkamp, MD, and Ofole Mgbako, MD

ABOUT THE AUTHORS

Robert Pitts and Angelica Cifuentes Kottkamp are with the Departments of Medicine and Infectious Diseases at New York University (NYU) Grossman School of Medicine and NYC Health + Hospitals/Bellevue, New York, NY. Ofole Mgbako is with the Departments of Medicine, Population Health, and Infectious Diseases at NYU Grossman School of Medicine and NYC Health + Hospitals/Bellevue.

See also Kennedy-Shaffer, p. 778, and Cope et al., p. 815.

After 40 years of efforts to address inequities in HIV prevention and treatment, one of the most useful tools to emerge is a framework for outlining prevention and treatment services—the HIV care continuum. Briefly, the care continuum is a framework that identifies the steps, or "bars," a person can take from time of HIV diagnosis, treatment initiation, and retention in care, to achieve viral suppression (https://bit.ly/3MPscEQ). Utilizing this framework can also elucidate the pressure points at each stage of the continuum where inequities persist, causing widening of gaps that prevent people from progressing successfully from testing to treatment. Public health practitioners can employ the care continuum framework to serve as a model for what could have been an equity-based approach to responding to COVID-19 and mpox and what should be an equity-based approach for future infectious disease outbreaks.

THE BAR BEFORE THE BARS

Our collective experience in understanding the barriers to ending the HIV epidemic in the United States has identified critical pathways that stigma in its multiple forms (e.g., racism, sexism, ageism, poverty, homophobia) can operate at each juncture of the care continuum to reduce successful health outcomes. The National Alliance of State and Territorial AIDS Directors has identified these multiple forms of stigma as the "bar before the bars" of the care continuum (https://nastad.org/issues/stigma). With respect to the mpox outbreak, stigma narratives shaped the public health response and policy decisions, as well as individual engagement with health care services. For example, provider refusal to take thorough sexual histories or physically examine patients increased patient distrust of providers and the health care system overall. These implicit and explicit forms of stigma were key drivers of delays in maximizing attainment of each stage of a care continuum: timely testing, diagnosis, and treatment. Recognizing the impact of stigma in all its forms is central to address inequities in care continuum outcomes and can be instructive in reducing barriers to address future outbreaks.

DELAYS IN TESTING

Initially in the mpox outbreak, limited testing availability impacted patients who were uninsured or underinsured or lacked a primary care doctor. As a consequence, many people went from emergency department to emergency department because providers did not initially recognize their lesions as mpox. Others were tested and experienced significant delays in diagnosis or were seen in clinical settings with no clear process for navigating patients to immediate treatment. Furthermore, in viral illnesses with skin manifestations, there is the possibility of underrecognition of disease in darker skin tones on the part of providers. It has been well documented that clinician inability to recognize certain diseases in darker skin tones may lead to differential clinical outcomes by race/ethnicity.[1] Among those ultimately tested and diagnosed, significant internalized or anticipated stigma concerns around disclosure to friends or partners may have limited contact tracing efforts as noted by Cope et al. (p. 815 in this issue of *AJPH*) despite its recognition as a key strategy for preventing the spread of infectious diseases in outbreak settings.[2]

DELAYS OBTAINING CARE AND TREATMENT

"Test-to-treat" strategies, commonly recognized as an HIV management approach, were also used for COVID-19 responses with the expansion of treatment options like nirmatrelvir/ritonavir. With mpox, delays from time of specimen collection to diagnosis combined with significant barriers to access tecovirimat (https://bit.ly/41CJHMF), the treatment option presumed effective against mpox, made a test-to-treat strategy nearly impossible. In New York City, mpox cases were also clustered among people experiencing homelessness and housing insecurity, as well as undocumented immigrants or low-wage workers, leaving these groups particularly vulnerable to delayed treatment initiation and preventable morbidity.

DELAYS IN ADEQUATE VACCINE COVERAGE

The initial criteria for access to JYNNEOS, the smallpox vaccine with presumed efficacy against mpox, was based on a person's sexual preference and number of partners. Early public health messaging that provided inaccurate and incomplete information gave a false sense of security to people who did not have multiple sexual partners or did not engage in specific sexual acts thereby potentially reducing early vaccination rates. Patients also described fear of being seen at mpox vaccination centers given the stress of being "outed" as a member of the lesbian, gay, bisexual, transgender, queer, or questioning (LGBTQ+) community or as someone with multiple sexual partners.

In addition, mpox vaccine roll-out in New York City was uneven at first, although it improved drastically once vaccine supplies were readily available. However, the initial New York City vaccine stockpile was far from adequate to administer to those at risk, forcing health care authorities to develop stringent eligibility criteria as described previously. Second, access to vaccine appointments was complex, time consuming, tech dependent, and poorly communicated across media outlets. As vaccine distribution strategies were enhanced given increased vaccine availability, vaccine eligibility criteria were relaxed (Kennedy-Shaffer, p. 778), and supplies were allocated to community-based organizations to distribute to already engaged clientele.[3] Thus, the confusing and, at times, contradictory messaging around vaccine eligibility as well as implications for those receiving vaccination may have also played a role in contact tracing becoming less efficient at identifying exposed contacts as noted by Cope et al.

MITIGATING THE HARMS OF STIGMA

These recent outbreaks have reinforced the need to diminish the impact of stigma early and rapidly. Educational outreach directed toward communities, policymakers, and health care workers may reduce experiences of stigma and enhance individual benefits and population-level effectiveness of interventions. In our own experience at NYC Health + Hospitals/Bellevue, we proactively provided frequent informational sessions to our staff covering the current status of the mpox outbreak and proper use of personal protective equipment, and highlighted the low risk of mpox transmissibility between patients and health care staff. We stressed how multiple forms of stigma, experienced both inside and outside care settings, could ultimately hinder timely testing, diagnosis, access to treatment, and vaccination.

FOSTERING AN EQUITY-FOCUSED CARE CONTINUUM

Our experiences with COVID-19 and mpox reinforce the need to increase access to health care for people who are uninsured, underinsured, or lack a primary care provider as early as possible during future outbreaks, as this is paramount to reduce inequities along the care continuum.

The following approaches can support the establishment of an equity-focused care continuum. First, with regard to testing availability, the CDC's Social Vulnerability Index (https://bit.ly/3KOlKvf) is a potential model that can be leveraged to determine allocation of early testing services. This approach prioritizes bringing new testing and diagnostic technology directly to those communities that are most vulnerable but also have the least access to care. Second, partnering with emergency departments early, given infected persons may access their services throughout the phases of an outbreak, is critical to ensure all persons are assessed appropriately and linked for treatment if indicated. Third, training medical providers to initiate treatment at the time of testing if clinical signs and symptoms are suggestive of mpox, especially among the groups with highest disease incidence, can minimize gaps in treatment uptake. Fourth, patient navigators can prove instrumental to optimize linkage after diagnosis and adherence to treatment. For vulnerable groups, such as persons experiencing homelessness, partnering with community-based organizations can enhance opportunities for linkages to services (e.g., food pantries, housing support) that can reduce inequities in social determinants of health that otherwise prevent marginalized persons from being retained in care. And, lastly, a robust telehealth service that can offer disease management support as well as referrals for additional resources (mental health care, food, shelter, and health care for their other medical conditions) may enhance and expand engagement in care.[4]

CONCLUSIONS

The 2022 mpox outbreak exemplified inequities in health care as infections were disproportionately concentrated among Black and Brown and LGBTQ+ communities (https://bit.ly/3AwjJiJ), with limited access to testing, treatment, and vaccinations. Our response to control future outbreaks of infectious diseases must be centered around an equity-based care continuum. The application of a holistic care continuum model for future outbreaks will permit active monitoring of an epidemic as it evolves, the reduction of various forms of stigma, and identification of populations in most need of further resources to enhance testing, treatment, and engagement in care. The success of such strategies relies on inclusive policy and committed funding. The critical lessons of mpox can set us up to equitably respond to the next infectious disease emergency, preventing unnecessary morbidity and mortality and building a public health practice of consequence. AJPH

CORRESPONDENCE

Correspondence should be sent to Robert Pitts, 462 First Ave, New York, NY 10016 (e-mail: robert.pitts@nyulangone.org). Reprints can be ordered at https://ajph.org by clicking the "Reprints" link.

PUBLICATION INFORMATION

Full Citation: Pitts RA, Cifuentes Kottkamp A, Mgbako O. An equity-focused care continuum framework for mpox and future infectious disease outbreaks: a public health of consequence, July 2023. *Am J Public Health*. 2023;113(7): 729–731.

Acceptance Date: April 22, 2023.

DOI: https://doi.org/10.2105/AJPH.2023.307326

CONTRIBUTIONS

All authors conceptualized and wrote the content of this article.

CONFLICTS OF INTEREST

The authors have no conflicts of interest to disclose.

REFERENCES

1. Buster KJ, Stevens EI, Elmets CA. Dermatologic health disparities. *Dermatol Clin*. 2012;30(1):53–59. https://doi.org/10.1016/j.det.2011.08.002
2. El-Sadr WM, Platt J, Bernitz M, Reyes M. Contact tracing: barriers and facilitators. *Am J Public Health*. 2022;112(7):1025–1033. https://doi.org/10.2105/AJPH.2022.306842
3. Holloway IW. Lessons for community-based scale-up of monkeypox vaccination from previous disease outbreaks among gay, bisexual, and other men who have sex with men in the United States. *Am J Public Health*. 2022;112(11):1572–1575. https://doi.org/10.2105/AJPH.2022.307075
4. Lo Piccolo AJ, Wallach A, McPherson TD, et al. The role of a tertiary level safety net hospital in New York City's 2022 mpox outbreak. *Health Secur*. 2023;21(2):146–155. https://doi.org/10.1089/hs.2022.0120

Looking Back: Decarcerating Immigration Prisons as a Tool for Improved Health

Caitlin Patler, PhD, Altaf Saadi, MD, MSc, and Ahilan Arulanantham, JD

ABOUT THE AUTHORS

Caitlin Patler is with the Department of Sociology, University of California, Davis. Altaf Saadi is with the Department of Neurology, Massachusetts General Hospital and Harvard Medical School, Boston. Ahilan Arulanantham is with the Center for Immigration Law & Policy, School of Law, University of California, Los Angeles.

Between 2008 and 2018, US Immigration and Customs Enforcement (ICE) apprehended more than two million noncitizens in the United States.[1] On any given day, ICE imprisons tens of thousands of such individuals in more than 200 jails or privately operated facilities under prisonlike conditions. Many imprisoned immigrants are held for years, with limited access to attorneys or other constitutional protections available under US criminal law. We refer to these facilities as "immigration prisons" because they have physical and legal characteristics of prisons and because immigrants experience them as imprisonment.

From the early days of the COVID-19 pandemic, academics, advocates, and imprisoned immigrants raised the alarm that immigration prisons could facilitate the vast spread of the virus, given the overcrowding, poor conditions of confinement, and grossly inadequate health care present in ICE's prison system,[2] coupled with ICE's historic unresponsiveness to violations of its own basic care standards.[3] They also warned that ICE's poor medical care could prove particularly dangerous during a pandemic, because many detained people have health conditions that create greater risk of poor COVID-19 outcomes.[4] Although ICE eventually put mitigation efforts in place, the monthly COVID-19 case rate among imprisoned immigrants between April and August 2020 was 5.7 to 21.8 times higher than that of the US general population during the same period.[5] The *Washington Post* editorial board labeled ICE "the superspreader agency."[6]

ICE's failure to prevent the spread of the virus ultimately proved deadly: on May 6, 2020, Carlos Escobar Mejia, a 57-year-old immigrant from El Salvador who had lived in the United States for 40 years, was the first known person to die of COVID-19 in ICE custody. Escobar Mejia's death, like many that followed, was entirely preventable. In their clear, evidence-based commentary in *AJPH* in January 2021,[7] a multidisciplinary team of researchers led by William D. Lopez emphasized that mass release would be the most effective way—perhaps the only way—to prevent the spread of COVID-19 infection and death in immigration prisons. The authors argued that ICE's purported in-facility mitigation efforts were some of the least effective ways to control outbreaks in congregate settings and that ICE's history of failing to "effectively implement [even] the most basic . . . controls"[7(p111)] would limit the success of any such efforts. Indeed, medical researchers subsequently showed that ICE's COVID-19 mitigation efforts significantly differed from Centers for Disease Control and Prevention guidelines regarding, for example, testing and isolation protocols.[8]

Release from detention, Lopez et al. argued, would be the safest and most humane solution to mitigate the spread of COVID-19 in immigration prisons. The authors cited guidelines for safe release into the community, which were developed by the Women's Refugee Commission, Physicians for Human Rights, and Freedom for Immigrants. Importantly, Lopez et al. distinguished their call for mass release from selective releases (which can be "inconsistent, arbitrary, and discriminatory") and deportation (which would be both "inhumane" and illegal if it circumvented established administrative legal processes).[7(p113)]

Lopez et al. was frequently cited by public health experts, advocates for detained people, and, perhaps most visibly, the World Health Organization in its August 2021 special focus on COVID-19 in prisons as evidence that "SARS-CoV-2 transmission and other health issues continue to be a challenge in prisons,"[9(p8)] despite mitigation measures.

CURRENT STATE OF KNOWLEDGE AND ACTION

The COVID-19 pandemic underscored the acute dangers of carceral settings such as immigration prisons, highlighting an urgent need for greater risk mitigation and decarceration more

AJPH July 2023, Vol 113, No. 7

generally. Lopez et al. provided an important entry point for those ongoing conversations. Since their article's publication at the end of 2020, several new peer-reviewed studies using multiple data sources have provided additional evidence of the extensive and systemic harms of immigration detention and how mass release could mitigate many of those harms in and outside the context of a pandemic. We now review some of this new work.

Recent research shows that ICE's response to the pandemic may have increased rather than mitigated health harms, as predicted by Lopez et al. An analysis of medical expert declarations from detention facilities in six US states in 2020 and 2021 found evidence of medical mismanagement and neglect of detained individuals.[10] Another study, analyzing ICE administrative data from 2018 to 2022, found a significant increase in ICE's use of solitary confinement during the pandemic, despite the practice being so harmful to mental health that the United Nations defines confinement longer than 15 days as torture.[11] A third study examined ICE administrative data to analyze sexual assault allegations and found that more than 70% of immigration prisons reported sexual assault allegations during the study period, with allegations against facility staff significantly increasing by 134% from 2019 to 2021.[12]

Recent research using data collected directly from detained immigrants underscores how conditions of imprisonment manifested in deleterious health consequences, even outside the context of the pandemic. An analysis of health survey data from detained immigrants in California found individual and cumulative associations between conditions of confinement and poor physical and mental health.[1] In another study using interview data from formerly detained immigrants in New York, immigrants perceived detention as "harmful by design" to their health and dignity.[13] That this health-harming system continues is especially problematic given strong evidence that imprisonment is unnecessary to accomplish its stated legal purpose of ensuring compliance with immigration legal proceedings.[14]

Recent research has also substantiated claims that the health harms of detention could be mitigated through release: in a panel study of individuals detained in California and then released into the community, participants reported fewer

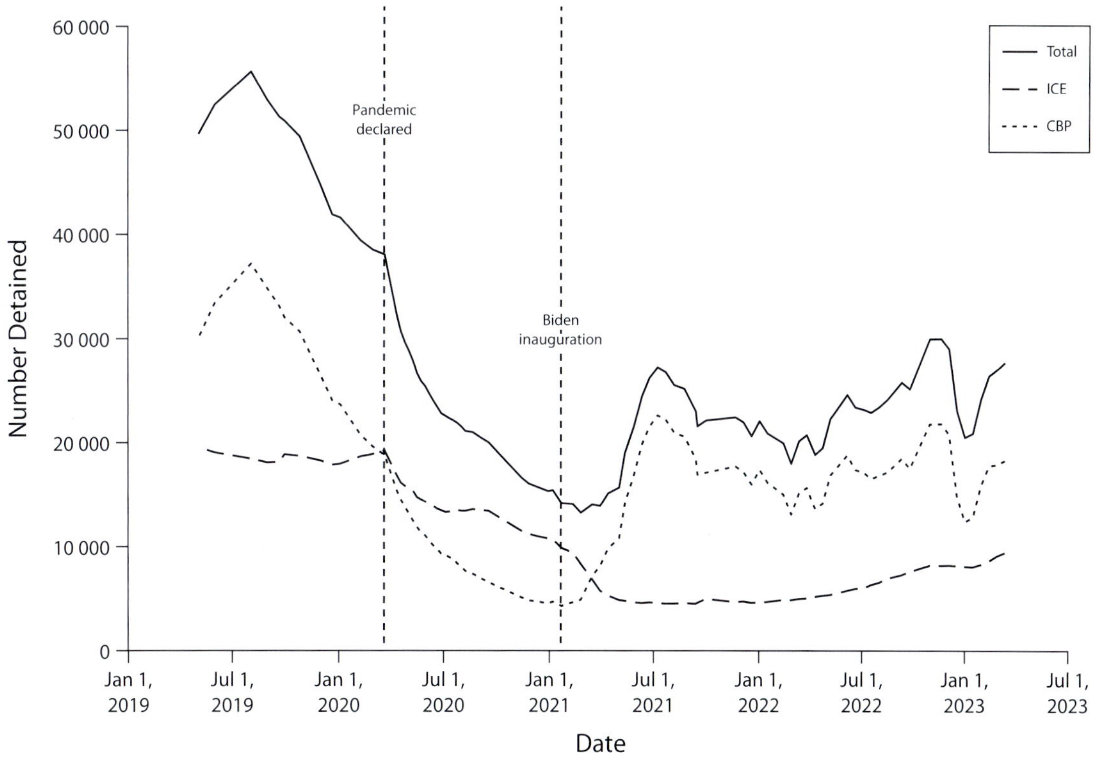

FIGURE 1— Number of People in ICE Custody by Arresting Agency: TRAC, United States, May 4, 2019–March 12, 2023

Note. CBP = Customs and Border Protection; ICE = US Immigration and Customs Enforcement; TRAC = Transactional Records Access Clearinghouse.
Source. Authors' tabulations of data from TRAC, https://trac.syr.edu/immigration/quickfacts/detention.html.

physical, psychological, and overall symptoms of stress, as well as improved general health after release from detention compared with during imprisonment.[15] These results provide promising evidence of the benefits of release.

ACTION TO MITIGATE HARM

Ongoing and future health research about immigration prisons can inform and be informed by efforts outside academia by detained people and their advocates. We now briefly highlight several ongoing efforts to expose ICE's inability to effectively control the pandemic in its facilities and push ICE to implement better mitigation efforts, which should include testing, vaccine access, and mass release.

In April 2020, a class of imprisoned immigrants at the largest ICE facility in California, the Adelanto ICE Processing Center, filed a lawsuit demanding that ICE release enough people to permit six-foot social distancing at all times, including when sleeping.[16] The district court initially ordered a substantial population reduction, but ICE appealed that order and won an interim ruling preventing it from going into effect. Several months later, a massive outbreak occurred at the facility: 66 people—58 imprisoned immigrants and eight staff members—tested positive in one week. Shortly afterward, in October 2020, the court of appeals ruled in the detained peoples' favor. The resulting release of several hundred people constituted the single largest population reduction at any immigration prison during the pandemic. The court's order remains in effect as of February 2023.

In March 2020, a group of prison civil rights lawyers filed a lawsuit demanding that ICE identify medically vulnerable imprisoned immigrants in its custody and then consider those individuals for release in light of their unique vulnerability during the pandemic. In the following months, the district court issued several orders that led to the release of medically vulnerable immigrants across the country. An appellate court reversed those orders in October 2021 but only after many releases occurred.[17] Numerous similar cases were filed throughout the country.

There have been other advocacy efforts as well, for example, attempts to push state and local health departments to take more aggressive steps to ensure that ICE pursued proper mitigation and vaccination efforts. Taken together, these efforts sought to save lives in the short term as part of longer-term goals to end the use of imprisonment in immigration legal proceedings altogether.

CONCLUSIONS

The population detained by ICE fell during the COVID-19 pandemic (Figure 1) to the lowest levels in 20 years, in large part because of the closure of the border to people seeking asylum, court-ordered mass releases such as those described herein, and interruptions to ICE field operations that limited new apprehensions. However, although the Biden administration has reduced funding for ICE detention beds,[18] beginning in 2021, ICE ramped up its operations once again, and the detained population has held steady between 20 000 and 30 000 people per day. This is largely driven by Customs and Border Protection arrests (Figure 1), which are likely to continue as the Biden administration expands Trump era programs limiting the admission of asylum seekers at the border.[19]

Advocates continue to make the case for decreased funding, and ultimately abolition, of the immigration prison system based on the extensive abuses in facilities and robust empirical evidence establishing that incarcerating immigrants is not necessary to ensure the functioning of immigration laws. In the interim, human rights attorneys continue to advocate improved facility conditions, such as decreasing reliance on solitary confinement, improving access to legal representation, and other reforms.

A robust body of research makes clear that immigration imprisonment is undeniably harmful—even deadly—for detained people. Importantly, health harms are not evenly distributed: recent research provides evidence that Black immigrants are overrepresented in punitive or harmful conditions in ICE facilities.[20] Additional research is needed to inform efforts to best protect the health of historically marginalized and vulnerable groups.

Public health professionals can continue to partner with legal professionals and community advocates to document the health harms of immigration prisons and call for a system that is responsive to scientific evidence and upholds human rights principles. This can include a radical reenvisioning of a structure designed to punish rather than heal.

The growing body of evidence is unequivocal: imprisoning immigrants is harmful to health and unnecessary for the operation of immigration legal proceedings. As long as mass incarceration remains a key strategy of immigration law enforcement, imprisoned people will continue to experience the health harms resulting from it. Congress can legislate an end to imprisonment in immigration legal proceedings. Indeed, many countries simply do not operate immigration prisons, and the United States itself did not do so for long periods of its history, including for several decades after World War II. The dismantling of this harmful system is critical to protecting health in and beyond the context of a global pandemic. AJPH

CORRESPONDENCE

Correspondence should be sent to Caitlin Patler, 1283 Social Sciences & Humanities, University of California, Davis, 1 Shields Ave, Davis, CA 95616 (e-mail: patler@ucdavis.edu). Reprints can be ordered at http://www.ajph.org by clicking the "Reprints" link.

PUBLICATION INFORMATION

Full Citation: Patler C, Saadi A, Arulanantham A. Looking back: decarcerating immigration prisons as a tool for improved health. *Am J Public Health*. 2023;113(7):732–735.

Acceptance Date: March 15, 2023.

DOI: https://doi.org/10.2105/AJPH.2023.307293

CONTRIBUTORS

C. Patler conceptualized the editorial, and all authors contributed to the writing.

ACKNOWLEDGMENTS

The authors thank the editors of *AJPH*.

CONFLICTS OF INTEREST

The authors have no conflicts of interest to disclose.

REFERENCES

1. Saadi A, Patler C, De Trinidad Young ME. Cumulative risk of immigration prison conditions on health outcomes among detained immigrants in California. *J Racial Ethn Health Disparities*. 2022; 9(6):2518–2532. https://doi.org/10.1007/s40615-021-01187-1
2. Patler C, Saadi A, Yazdan-Panah H. Immigrant detention, COVID-19, and opportunities for action. Available at: https://globalmigration.ucdavis.edu/immigrant-detention-covid-19-and-opportunities-action. Accessed February 16, 2023.
3. Department of Homeland Security, Office of Inspector General. Concerns about ICE detainee treatment and care at four detention facilities. Available at: https://www.oig.dhs.gov/sites/default/files/assets/2019-06/OIG-19-47-Jun19.pdf. Accessed February 16, 2023.
4. Patler C, Saadi A. Risk of poor outcomes with COVID-19 among US detained immigrants: a cross-sectional study. *J Immigr Minor Health*. 2021;23(4):863–866. https://doi.org/10.1007/s10903-021-01173-z
5. Erfani P, Uppal N, Lee CH, Mishori R, Peeler KR. COVID-19 testing and cases in immigration detention centers, April–August 2020. *JAMA*. 2021;325(2):182–184. https://doi.org/10.1001/jama.2020.21473
6. Editorial Board. ICE is the superspreader agency. *Washington Post*. May 2, 2021. Available at: https://www.washingtonpost.com/opinions/ice-is-the-superspreader-agency/2021/05/01/eb079944-a9f2-11eb-8c1a-56f0cb4ff3b5_story.html. Accessed March 26, 2023.
7. Lopez WD, Kline N, LeBrón A, et al. Preventing the spread of COVID-19 in immigration detention centers requires the release of detainees. *Am J Public Health*. 2021;111(1):110–115. https://doi.org/10.2105/AJPH.2020.305968
8. Openshaw JJ, Travassos MA. COVID-19 outbreaks in US immigrant detention centers: the urgent need to adopt CDC guidelines for prevention and evaluation. *Clin Infect Dis*. 2021;72(1):153–154. https://doi.org/10.1093/cid/ciaa692
9. World Health Organization. COVID-19 weekly epidemiological update. August 17, 2021. Available at: https://apps.who.int/iris/bitstream/handle/10665/344324/CoV-weekly-sitrep17Aug21-eng.pdf?sequence=1&isAllowed=y. Accessed March 26, 2023.
10. Zeidan AJ, Goodall H, Sieben A, Parmar P, Burner E. Medical mismanagement in Southern US immigration and customs enforcement detention facilities: a thematic analysis of secondary medical records. *J Immigr Minor Health*. [Online ahead of print January 30, 2023]. https://doi.org/10.1007/s10903-023-01451-y
11. Nwadiuko J, Nishi A, Terp S, Dekker AM, Bustamante AV, Parmar P. Solitary confinement use in immigration detention before and after the beginning of the SARS-CoV-2 pandemic. *J Gen Intern Med*. [Epub ahead of print February 7, 2023]. https://doi.org/10.1007/s11606-023-08055-0
12. Lue N, Nwadiuko J, Parmar P, Zeidan A. Trends in sexual assault against detainees in US immigration detention centers, 2018–2022. *JAMA*. 2023;329(4):338–339. https://doi.org/10.1001/jama.2022.22938
13. Diaz C, Ortiz V, Sanchez L, et al. Harmful by design—a qualitative study of the health impacts of immigration detention. *J Gen Intern Med*. [Epub ahead of print November 30, 2022]. https://doi.org/10.1007/s11606-022-07914-6
14. Eagly I, Shafer S. Measuring *in absentia* removal in immigration court. *Univ Pa Law Rev*. 2020; 168(4):817–876.
15. Patler C, Saadi A. Young MEdT, Franco K. Release from US immigration detention may improve physical and psychological stress and health: results from a two-wave panel study in California. *SSM - Ment Health (Lond)*. 2021;1:100035. https://doi.org/10.1016/j.ssmmh.2021.100035
16. *Roman v. Wolf*, 977 F.3d 935 (9th Cir. 2020).
17. *Fraihat v. US ICE*, 16 F.4th 613 (9th Cir. 2021).
18. *New York Times*. Biden to ask Congress for 9,000 fewer immigration detention beds. March 25, 2022. Available at: https://www.nytimes.com/2022/03/25/us/politics/biden-immigration-detention-beds.html. Accessed March 26, 2023.
19. Department of Homeland Security, US Citizenship and Immigration Services. Proposed rule: circumvention of lawful pathways. *Fed Reg*. 2023; 88(36):11704–11752.
20. Franco K, Patler C, Reiter K. Punishing status and the punishment status quo: solitary confinement in US immigration prisons, 2013–2017. *Punishm Soc*. 2021;24(2):170–195. https://doi.org/10.1177/1462474520967804

Looking Back: How the COVID-19 Pandemic Provided Opportunity to Equitably Improve Meal Provision

Chelsea R. Singleton, PhD, MPH, and Gabriella M. McLoughlin, PhD, MS

ABOUT THE AUTHORS

Chelsea R. Singleton is with the Department of Social, Behavioral, and Population Sciences, Tulane School of Public Health and Tropical Medicine, New Orleans, LA. Gabriella M. McLoughlin is with the Department of Kinesiology, Temple University College of Public Health, Philadelphia, PA.

AJPH July 2023, Vol 113, No. 7

The onset of the COVID-19 pandemic in 2020 resulted in unprecedented disruptions to every social and economic facet of life.[1] By March 2020, increased case rates and state-mandated stay-at-home orders prompted the closure of public schools in all 50 states and territories of the United States.[2] For schools with large populations of low-income students who participate in the National School Lunch Program and the School Breakfast Program, school administrators and staff expressed great concern regarding potential increases in food insecurity rates among students.[1,3] Children and adolescents that received meals from these programs during school hours no longer had access to this important resource.

In November 2020, Kinsey et al. published an original analytic essay in the *American Journal of Public Health* that (1) described the negative impact of school closures on school meal delivery and (2) summarized innovative strategies implemented nationally and locally to address the disruption in school meal provision.[4] In this editorial, we reflect on the Kinsey et al. article, which garnered significant media attention in the United States and abroad following its publication. In addition, we provide our thoughts on the potential impact of their work on research, practice, and policy aimed at equitably improving meal delivery in various settings.

A SHOCK TO THE SYSTEM

Prior to the pandemic, schools were a critical part of the food and nutrition safety net for American families.[3] More than 30 million school-aged children participate in the National School Lunch Program and roughly 15 million participate in the School Breakfast Program.[5,6] Collectively, these programs provide free meals (eligibility: household income < 130% of poverty level as determined by the US Census Bureau) or reduced-price meals (eligibility: household income < 185% of poverty level) to students every day to mitigate risk of food insecurity.[5,6] As schools ceased in-person instruction in response to rising COVID-19 infection rates, millions of children lost access to a stable source of nutrition assistance, which resulted in significant increases in food insecurity rates among children and adolescents.[3]

This nationwide disruption in school meal delivery was an unforeseen challenge that many school districts were not prepared to address.[4,7] Prior to the onset of the pandemic, there was limited understanding of how school meal service would respond in the event of a nationwide disruption persisting for many months.[7] Schools immediately started pivoting to alternative models of meal service, which included serving school meals under the Seamless Summer Option or the Summer Food Service Program.[4] Unfortunately, some parameters governing these provisions (e.g., meals must be consumed on the school site, students must be present to receive meals, only one meal can be served at a time) presented logistical issues incongruent with the nature of a pandemic.[4,7] These challenges necessitated a series of waivers from the US Department of Agriculture (USDA), which allowed schools to serve meals with greater flexibility.[4] Studies conducted to examine state, territory, and jurisdiction responses to these waivers highlighted the rapid-cycle dissemination efforts by authorities to provide implementation guidance to school districts and up-to-date communications on meal pickup sites to families.[7,8]

In the early stages of transition to more flexible models of meal delivery, schools and districts reported low participation.[4] Accordingly, Kinsey et al. undertook a rapid-cycle study to estimate the magnitude of the problem, and thus calculate the number of meals not served ("missed") because of the transition from in-person to socially distanced meal provision.[4] Their analyses of national data provided a figure of 1.15 billion missed meals due to school closures.[4] This number was staggering and naturally caught the attention of several news outlets (n = 48) who issued press releases (n = 63) on this research.[9] Such media attention was paralleled by scientific publications (n = 79 to date) that cited the article for the purpose of (1) highlighting calls to action related to food insecurity, (2) studying food insecurity–related issues exacerbated by the COVID-19 pandemic, or (3) introducing relevant cross-sectional or intervention research conducted in local, national, or international settings.[9] It is clear the Kinsey et al. article underscored major challenges and much-needed innovations in meal service for schools in the early months of the pandemic.[4] These innovations may prove to be relevant to endeavors aimed at improving meal delivery in other community settings.

WORKING OUT THE KINKS

Despite describing several innovations in school meal provision, the Kinsey et al. article revealed gaps in knowledge and unanswered questions regarding the efficacy and feasibility of meal delivery.[4] These questions and gaps present opportunities for researchers, practitioners, federal policymakers, and communities to (1) reflect on the challenges and successes associated with the COVID-19 pandemic and (2) identify targeted areas for improvement. In doing so, future food assistance efforts will build on lessons learned and implement strategies in an equitable manner.[8]

First, research is needed to critically assess the efficacy of the federal waiver rollout process. The Kinsey et al. article highlighted how early COVID-19 legislation, such as the Families First Coronavirus Response Act, gave the USDA authority to grant waivers to states so they can alter how school meals are delivered.[4] Acting fast during emergencies is essential to ensuring that children and families are provided support in a timely manner. The first few nationwide waivers (granted in March 2020) addressed major practical concerns by allowing schools to offer families flexible meal service times, multiple meals at once in the same day, and varied delivery options (e.g., grab-and-go, curbside pick-up, home delivery).[4,7] However, waivers issued in the following months addressed systemic concerns by relaxing policies related to eligibility criteria and reimbursement rules for meals that do not meet nutritional requirements.[4] To our knowledge, there is a dearth of data on the efficacy and acceptability of the waiver rollout process. This research is necessary to determine how well the rollout timeline and order were received by important stakeholders such as school administrators, cafeteria staff, and food suppliers. In addition, this work will identify potential waivers that should be considered in the future. Kinsey et al. mentioned that the USDA does not reimburse for travel expenses associated with home delivery of meals.[4] Given the resource accessibility issues that often affect rural and blighted urban areas,[10] federal policymakers should consider this and other issues facing disadvantaged populations.

Second, more research is needed to determine the role of key socioenvironmental factors in the design and implementation of meal delivery programs. The meal delivery strategies implemented by some schools during the pandemic, particularly those in urban areas, raised questions concerning transportation, public safety, and discrimination.[8,11–13] These socioenvironmental factors should be considered when developing novel strategies to equitably improve school meal delivery and meal delivery in other settings.[8,14] Prior research has linked insufficient public and personal transportation to adverse nutritional outcomes, such as food insecurity, in communities with low access to healthy food retailers (e.g., supermarkets, grocery stores).[11] Perceptions of personal safety and discrimination can affect the food shopping patterns and decision-making of consumers, which include retailer choice.[12,13] Socially and economically disadvantaged populations, such as low-income individuals and people of color, are more likely to report experiences of discrimination and reside in communities with high crime rates and poor public transportation options.[11–13] Therefore, it is important to consider these, and other relevant social determinants of health, if the ultimate goal of strategy development is to foster equity across communities and populations.

THE FUTURE IS HERE

The findings and recommendations presented in the Kinsey et al. article suggest that the COVID-19 pandemic has provided researchers, practitioners, and policymakers with an opportunity to improve meal provision efforts in schools and other community settings.[4] Improving meal provision, particularly those programs serving socially and economically disadvantaged populations, will strengthen the food safety net in communities across the country.[14,15] In addition to the innovative strategies described by Kinsey et al., individuals and organizations who hold decision-making power should consider

(1) encouraging the adoption of Community Eligibility Provision (CEP), (2) facilitating sustainable public school–academic institution partnerships, and (3) engaging communities and families in the strategy design and implementation processes.[14,15] Adoption of CEP by schools and school districts will allow students with fluctuating incomes to have access to meals, which provides a healthier school meal model for low-income and economically diverse communities.[15] Sustainable partnerships between public schools and academic institutions will facilitate the collection and analysis of real-time data on determinants of school meal implementation and uptake, leveraging the expertise of practitioners and the evaluation support of researchers. And finally, engaging community members, leaders, and families will allow organizations that provide meals to develop and introduce more effective and acceptable strategies. As the field continues to study the pandemic's impact on nutrition, health, and well-being, it is important to reflect on how lessons learned can lead to equitable improvements to public health. AJPH

CORRESPONDENCE

Correspondence should be sent to Chelsea R. Singleton, Assistant Professor, Department of Social, Behavioral, and Population Sciences, Tulane School of Public Health & Tropical Medicine, 1440 Canal St, Suite 2200-20, New Orleans, LA 70112 (e-mail: csingle1@tulane.edu). Reprints can be ordered at http://www.ajph.org by clicking the "Reprints" link.

PUBLICATION INFORMATION

Full Citation: Singleton CR, McLoughlin GM. Looking back: how the COVID-19 pandemic provided opportunity to equitably improve meal provision. *Am J Public Health.* 2023;113(7):736–738.

Acceptance Date: March 15, 2023.

DOI: https://doi.org/10.2105/AJPH.2023.307294

CONTRIBUTORS

Both C. R. Singleton and G. M. McLoughlin conceptualized this article, contributed to the writing, and approved the final version.

ACKNOWLEDGMENTS

We acknowledge Eliza Kinsey and her research team who published the article "School Closures During COVID-19: Opportunities for Innovation in Meal Service" in the November 2020 issue of *AJPH*.

CONFLICTS OF INTEREST

The authors have no conflicts of interest to declare.

REFERENCES

1. Pereira M, Oliveria AM. Poverty and food insecurity may increase as the threat of COVID-19 spreads. *Public Health Nutr.* 2020;23(17):3236–3240. https://doi.org/10.1017/S1368980020003493
2. Krishnamachari B, Morris A, Zastrow D, Dsida A, Harper B, Santella AJ. The role of mask mandates, stay at home orders and school closure in curbing the COVID-19 pandemic prior to vaccination. *Am J Infect Control.* 2021;49(8):1036–1042. https://doi.org/10.1016/j.ajic.2021.02.002
3. Wolfson JA, Leung CW. Food insecurity during COVID-19: an acute crisis with long-term health implications. *Am J Public Health.* 2020;110(12):1763–1765. https://doi.org/10.2105/AJPH.2020.305953
4. Kinsey EW, Hecht AA, Dunn CG, et al. School closures during COVID-19: opportunities for innovation in meal service. *Am J Public Health.* 2020;110(11):1635–1643. https://doi.org/10.2105/AJPH.2020.305875
5. US Dept of Agriculture, Food & Nutrition Service. The National School Lunch Program. Available at: https://fns-prod.azureedge.us/sites/default/files/resource-files/NSLPFactSheet.pdf. Accessed February 7, 2023.
6. US Dept of Agriculture, Food & Nutrition Service. The School Breakfast Program. Available at: https://fns-prod.azureedge.us/sites/default/files/resource-files/SBPfactsheet.pdf. Accessed February 7, 2023.
7. McLoughlin GM, Fleischhacker S, Hecht AA, et al. Feeding students during COVID-19–related school closures: a nationwide assessment of initial responses. *J Nutr Educ Behav.* 2020;52(12):1120–1130. https://doi.org/10.1016/j.jneb.2020.09.018
8. McLoughlin GM, McCarthy JA, McGuirt JT, Singleton CR, Gunn CG, Gadhoke P. Addressing food insecurity through a health equity lens: a case study of large urban school districts during the COVID-19 pandemic. *J Urban Health.* 2020;97(6):759–775. https://doi.org/10.1007/s11524-020-00476-0
9. American Public Health Association. Article metrics: school closures during COVID-19: opportunities for innovation in meal service. Available at: https://apha.altmetric.com/details/90540199/news. Accessed January 17, 2023.
10. Walker RE, Keane CR, Burke JG. Disparities and access to healthy food in the United States: a review of food deserts literature. *Health Place.* 2010;16(5):876–884. https://doi.org/10.1016/j.healthplace.2010.04.013
11. Bartfeld JS, Ryu JH, Wang L. Local characteristics are linked to food insecurity among households with elementary school children. *J Hunger Environ Nutr.* 2010;5(4):471–483. https://doi.org/10.1080/19320248.2010.527278
12. Cannuscio CC, Hillier A, Karpyn A, Glanz K. The social dynamics of healthy food shopping and store choice in an urban environment. *Soc Sci Med.* 2014;122:13–20. https://doi.org/10.1016/j.socscimed.2014.10.005
13. Zenk SN, Schulz AJ, Israel BA, et al. Food shopping behaviours and exposure to discrimination. *Public Health Nutr.* 2014;17(5):1167–1176. https://doi.org/10.1017/S136898001300075X
14. McLoughlin GM, Walsh-Bailey C, Singleton CR, Turner L. Investigating implementation of school health policies through a health equity lens: a measures development study protocol. *Front Public Health.* 2022;10:984130. https://doi.org/10.3389/fpubh.2022.984130
15. Hecht AA, Olarte DA, McLoughlin GM, Cohen JFW. Promising strategies to increase student participation in school meals. Healthy Eating Research. Issue Brief, November 2022. Available at: https://healthyeatingresearch.org/wp-content/uploads/2022/11/HER-Meal-Participation-Brief_final.pdf. Accessed January 17, 2023.

How Green Spaces Can Combat Gun Violence in America

John E. Dobbs, MPH, and Joseph V. Sakran, MD, MPH, MPA

ABOUT THE AUTHORS

John E. Dobbs is a medical student at The George Washington University, Washington, DC. Joseph V. Sakran is Vice Chair of Clinical Operations, Department of Surgery, Johns Hopkins Hospital, Baltimore, MD.

It has long been known that bustling cityscapes—and the people who occupy them—benefit from well-designed and maintained parks. Concrete, meet grass. Building, meet tree. The thought alone helps us breathe more deeply. People in the United States have benefited from urban parks since Frederick Law Olmsted, the nation's most famous landscape architect, orchestrated the construction of New York City's Central Park more than a century ago. But there is one benefit, in particular, that is both powerful and underrecognized: green spaces can reduce gun violence.

UNDERSTANDING THE RELATIONSHIP

It may be hard to conceptualize how green spaces have a direct effect on gun violence, yet the scientific literature is increasingly demonstrating this to be true. A robust systematic review[1] found that communities with more vegetation suffer from less crime in general, and although socioeconomic factors were not accounted for, green spaces had a particularly strong impact on reducing gun violence. In terms of controlling for the sociodemographic factors of income, rates of poverty, age, and level of education, a study out of Philadelphia, Pennsylvania,[2] found that greening previously abandoned lots not only reduced gun violence but also produced a significant positive economic impact on the criminal justice system: greening each abandoned lot yielded about $43 000 in savings. Additionally, remediating the vacant buildings in an area led to a statistically significant 39% reduction in firearm assaults.

Although further evaluation is required to fully understand both the multifaceted relationship and the direction of causality between public parks and public safety, we know that well-kept green spaces mitigate many of the precipitating factors leading to episodes of gun violence. Green spaces can reduce stress[1] and improve the mental health of nearby residents.[3] They also support the entire community by storing excess rainwater, cleaning the air, and reducing the urban heat island effect.[1,3,4] The reduced temperatures alone can lead to decreased episodes of aggression.[5]

Green spaces are also thought to have an effect on the social fabric of a community, contributing to the busy streets theory,[6] which identifies the factors that improve social cohesion in a neighborhood while also reducing violence. Civic pride, residential engagement, and activity in public are all key attributes of thriving communities. Green spaces support the busy streets theory because it gives people a place to congregate and something to take care of. With more foot traffic comes more opportunities for members of the community to be on the watch for any illicit activity, decreasing its likelihood to occur in that area. These attributes are also aligned with the third-generation iteration of crime prevention through environmental design, which is a method of crime reduction that focuses on decreasing crime rates by making spaces more livable in general.[7]

CURRENT SHORTFALLS

Although green spaces can yield many benefits, communities with the greatest need for green space receive the least of it. These "nongreen" communities are more likely to have residents that identify as low-income and Black or Latinx. These neighborhoods also often have the highest levels of gun violence. Compared with their White counterparts, Black children and adolescents are more than 13 times as likely to be victims of gun homicide.[8] Latinx adolescents and children suffer from gun homicide at roughly twice the rate as White children of the same age. To make matters worse, 2021 homicide rates were nearly 40% higher than 2019 numbers,[9] and these same Black and Latinx communities are likely bearing the brunt of this epidemic.

The collateral effects of this increased carnage may take multiple forms. From diverting limited hospital resources to sowing more unrest in the community, gun violence continues to be a disruptive force that has thus far proven difficult to shake. New tactics need to be deployed to prevent these tragedies from occurring in the first place. As professionals in public health and medicine, we recognize the need for an evidence-based approach as we tackle some of the most complex public health problems, such as gun violence.

One such solution should be to green the communities suffering from high rates of gun violence. In many cases, communities with high rates of gun violence have a surfeit of vacant or underdeveloped lots that are ripe for this type of investment. In their current form, these abandoned spaces are inhospitable for most forms of recreation and are ideal locations for criminal activity, which in turn increases the risk of gun violence. If a green intervention took place, many of the concepts outlined by the busy streets theory could take form. New parks present new opportunities for community members to engage in recreation. As more local residents engage in these spaces, there is not only a greater degree of social cohesion but also more opportunity for community member surveillance of illicit and violence-prone activity. This greater degree of surveillance will serve as a strong disincentive for this sort of activity in the future.

There are good examples of green investment taking root around the country. The High Line Network has brought innovative green spaces to cities such as New York; Philadelphia; Dallas, Texas; and Atlanta, Georgia.[10] One of the best cases of this network in action is in Washington, DC, which is building a new bridge and corresponding park adjacent to the historically Black neighborhood of Anacostia.[11] As these spaces develop, we will have more opportunities to measure their impact on gun violence.

THINKING CREATIVELY

Green space projects are not without criticism: some decry them for their capacity to spur gentrification. These concerns are well validated. Projects from the Highline in New York to the Beltline in Atlanta have made housing unaffordable for nearby residents.[11] However, green spaces are valuable and essential investments in communities that have long been left out of the green movements, such as those started by Olmsted. Green spaces must be implemented in a way that supports the intended community without making the surrounding area unaffordable, and people undertaking current projects are learning from the mistakes of their predecessors. The 11th Street Bridge Park in Anacostia is currently set to spend nearly half of its $177 million[11] budget on initiatives that directly combat gentrification, including affordable housing and training the nearby workforce. The park also has active input from the community through its land trust, and this input helps the project leaders effectively identify where and how to allocate funds.

Similarly, Friends of the Rail Park, a nonprofit in Philadelphia, is creating an equitable development plan to better support the surrounding community of the Philadelphia Rail Park, which is a project rehabilitating an unused railway in the city (Figure 1).[12] With foresight, community engagement, and thoughtful allocation of capital, green spaces can be created while minimizing the gentrifying effects of its presence.

There is no silver bullet for reducing gun violence in low-income communities,

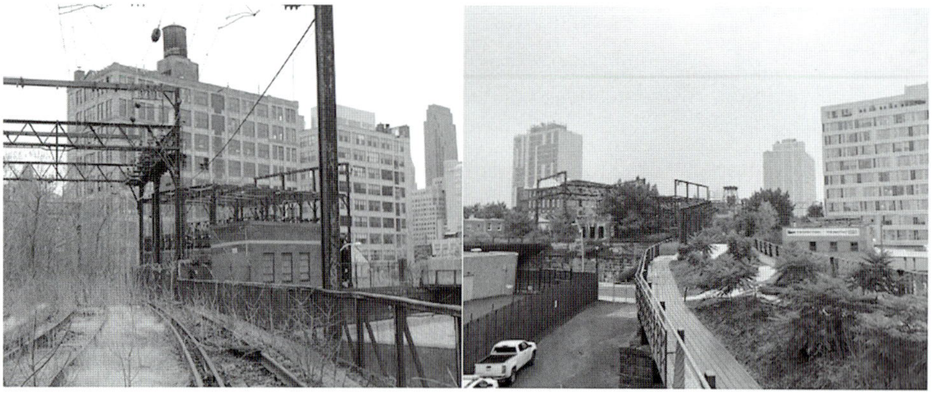

FIGURE 1— Philadelphia, Pennsylvania, Rail Park, Before and After Development: 2005, 2018

Source. Eric Cronin (March 26, 2005). Reading Viaduct in Philadelphia [Photograph]. Wikimedia Commons, https://commons.wikimedia.org/wiki/File:Reading_Viaduct.jpg#filehistory; airbus777 (October 8, 2018). The Rail Park, Philadelphia [Photograph]. Flickr, https://www.flickr.com/photos/erussell1984/44508073474/in/photostream.

particularly as they struggle against historical injustices such as redlining and persistent structural inequities in health care and education. This intractable problem requires a wide array of solutions, and one such solution should be investing in green infrastructure in these communities. Municipalities, small and large, should take advantage of President Biden's infrastructure bill,[13] which provides $21 billion to clean up historically polluted spaces across the country, a disproportionate number of which are in low-income communities of color. If deployed thoughtfully through new public green spaces, this investment could significantly reduce gun violence, yield positive returns for decades to come, and right many of the wrongs left by urban renewal.

HOW TO GET INVOLVED

There are still challenges to implementing these measures. City planners across the nation are already competing for the limited funding available to green these spaces that have long been ignored by society, and they could use the support of their respective local health care communities to achieve these goals. Engaging with city leadership can facilitate the creation of these vital green spaces. Using our clinical and investigational background, leaders in medical and public health research can delve into the relationship between green space and gun violence, which would generate the data required to understand this connection and provide a roadmap to building and maintaining safer communities. Even a social media post can help raise the profile of this important cause.

Leaders in medical and public health research concerned with the unmitigated rise in gun violence can and should use their expertise and credibility to support the greening of cities they live in. Although creating more parks is not a panacea for gun violence prevention, it is part of the solution to tackling this uniquely American public health problem. AJPH

CORRESPONDENCE

Correspondence should be sent to John E. Dobbs, The George Washington University School of Medicine and Health Sciences, 2300 I St NW, Washington, DC 20052 (e-mail: wyndobbs@gwu.edu). Reprints can be ordered at http://www.ajph.org by clicking the "Reprints" link.

PUBLICATION INFORMATION

Full Citation: Dobbs JE, Sakran JV. How green spaces can combat gun violence in America. *Am J Public Health*. 2023;113(7):739–741.

Acceptance Date: March 28, 2023.

DOI: https://doi.org/10.2105/AJPH.2023.307309

CONTRIBUTORS

J. E. Dobbs gathered the data for this editorial. Both authors drafted and edited the editorial.

CONFLICTS OF INTEREST

We have no conflicts of interest to disclose.

REFERENCES

1. Shepley M, Sachs N, Sadatsafavi H, Fournier C, Peditto K. The impact of green space on violent crime in urban environments: an evidence synthesis. *Int J Environ Res Public Health.* 2019;16(24):5119. https://doi.org/10.3390/ijerph16245119
2. Branas CC, Kondo MC, Murphy SM, South EC, Polsky D, MacDonald JM. Urban blight remediation as a cost-beneficial solution to firearm violence. *Am J Public Health.* 2016;106(12):2158–2164. https://doi.org/10.2105/AJPH.2016.303434
3. South EC, Hohl BC, Kondo MC, MacDonald JM, Branas CC. Effect of greening vacant land on mental health of community-dwelling adults: a cluster randomized trial. *JAMA Netw Open.* 2018;1(3):e180298. https://doi.org/10.1001/jamanetworkopen.2018.0298
4. Gibbens S. As the climate crisis worsens, cities turn to parks. *Natl Geogr.* May 21, 2019. Available at: https://www.nationalgeographic.com/environment/article/climate-crisis-cities-turn-to-parks. Accessed January 29, 2023.
5. Anderson CA. Temperature and aggression: ubiquitous effects of heat on occurrence of human violence. *Psychol Bull.* 1989;106(1):74–96. https://doi.org/10.1037/0033-2909.106.1.74
6. Aiyer SM, Zimmerman MA, Morrel-Samuels S, Reischl TM. From broken windows to busy streets: a community empowerment perspective. *Health Educ Behav.* 2015;42(2):137–147. https://doi.org/10.1177/1090198114558590
7. Mihinjac M, Saville G. Third-generation crime prevention through environmental design (CPTED). *Soc Sci.* 2019;8(6):182. https://doi.org/10.3390/socsci8060182
8. Kravitz-Wirtz N, Bruns A, Aubel AJ, Zhang X, Buggs SA. Inequities in community exposure to deadly gun violence by race/ethnicity, poverty, and neighborhood disadvantage among youth in large US cities. *J Urban Health.* 2022;99(4):610–625. https://doi.org/10.1007/s11524-022-00656-0
9. Lopez G. A violent crisis. *New York Times.* April 17, 2022. Available at: https://www.nytimes.com/2022/04/17/briefing/violent-crime-ukraine-war-week-ahead.html. Accessed October 14, 2022.
10. Schmidt G. Bringing nature back to the urban core. *New York Times.* February 12, 2019. Available at: https://www.nytimes.com/2019/02/12/business/cities-parks-green-space.html. Accessed November 19, 2022.
11. Kimble M, Wagner AD. Can Anacostia build a bridge without displacing its people? *New York Times.* August 9, 2022. Available at: https://www.nytimes.com/interactive/2022/08/09/headway/anacostia-bridge.html. Accessed November 19, 2022.
12. Schmidt S. "Who's benefiting?" As Chinatown gentrifies, rail park begins equitable development plan. February 24, 2022. Available at: https://nextcity.org/urbanist-news/whos-benefiting-as-chinatown-gentrifies-rail-park-begins-equitable-developm. Accessed January 26, 2023.
13. White House. The bipartisan infrastructure deal boosts clean energy jobs, strengthens resilience, and advances environmental justice. November 8, 2021. Available at: https://www.whitehouse.gov/briefing-room/statements-releases/2021/11/08/fact-sheet-the-bipartisan-infrastructure-deal-boosts-clean-energy-jobs-strengthens-resilience-and-advances-environmental-justice. Accessed March 31, 2023.

Veteran Truckers, the Supply Chain, and the Metabolic Syndrome: A Convergence of Crises

Michael A. Dunn, MD, Elliot B. Tapper, MD, and Shari S. Rogal, MD

ABOUT THE AUTHORS

Michael A. Dunn is with the Veterans Administration Northern Indiana Health Care System, Fort Wayne, and the Departments of Medicine and Biomedical Informatics, University of Pittsburgh, Pittsburgh, PA. Elliot B. Tapper is with the Veterans Administration Ann Arbor Health Care System, Ann Arbor, MI, and the Department of Medicine, University of Michigan, Ann Arbor. Shari S. Rogal is with the Center for Health Equity, Research and Promotion, Veterans Administration Pittsburgh Health Care System, Pittsburgh, PA, and the Department of Medicine, University of Pittsburgh.

AJPH July 2023, Vol 113, No. 7

The COVID-19 pandemic has exacerbated and highlighted gaps in the US supply chain, including a critical shortfall of truckers (i.e., those holding a commercial driver's license [CDL]). In response, in April 2022 the White House launched a government, industry, union, and veterans service organization collaboration, Task Force Movement, to recruit 80 000 veterans into the trucking industry.[1] Ten percent of employed US veterans already work as truckers, and many veterans complete their military service with the capacity and skills to succeed in the industry. As physicians for veterans, we believe that Task Force Movement's initiative to recruit new veteran truckers to improve the supply chain crisis presents an important opportunity to synchronize the effort with strong action to mitigate truckers' health risks from a second American crisis, the metabolic syndrome.

The cardiovascular, endocrine, hepatic, and renal complications of the metabolic syndrome are especially prevalent and severe among truckers. Two thirds of truckers are obese, and the majority have the additional metabolic risk factors of sedentary activity; long, stressful work hours; little sleep; and high-salt, high-fat diets.[2,3] The life expectancy of unionized US male truckers in 2000 was 61.3 years (vs 73.2 years for all US men), with ischemic heart disease as the leading cause of excess mortality.[4] If this reported premature mortality were to remain unchanged, the 80 000 new veteran truckers being recruited today would face a loss of 952 000 life-years.

To mitigate the health risks of trucking in general, and specifically to ensure that veterans are not put at greater risk by becoming truckers, it is critical to provide them with the tools to engage in preemptive, effective risk assessment and mitigation. Risk mitigation is a well-defined and widely taught military practice that most veterans have routinely used during their service to ensure health protection and mission success.[5] We believe that improved trucker health and risk mitigation require taking a series of specific actions in occupational health, public health policy, and education and advocacy.

OCCUPATIONAL HEALTH

Truckers enter their occupation by earning a CDL. At present, the medical standards set by the Federal Motor Carrier Safety Administration for CDL licensure are focused on drivers' ability to safely operate a vehicle and on their lack of disqualifying problems such as illicit substance use, uncontrolled diabetes, hypertension, and seizure risk.[6]

The CDL medical standards should be upgraded to provide drivers with an actionable, personalized profile of their occupational metabolic health risk derived from (1) a subjective assessment of sleep, physical activity, smoking, and diet; (2) an objective examination of body mass index, blood pressure, and physical capacity with gait speed and handgrip strength[7]; and (3) blood testing for known predictors of cardiovascular risk (low-density lipoprotein cholesterol), diabetes complications (hemoglobin A1C), kidney function (urinalysis and creatinine), and risk for progression of fatty liver disease (FIB-4 index, calculated from age, aspartate and alanine aminotransferases, and platelet count).[8] Newly qualified CDL holders should meet with a CDL medical examiner to review specific health improvement recommendations derived from a standardized predictive risk model, such as a patient-specific model with personalized decision paths.[9]

STRUCTURE AND POLICY

In addition to focusing on individual truckers, structural and policy actions are needed to improve trucker population health by supporting ease of access to healthy food options at truck stops, providing cost-free nicotine replacement therapy for smokers, and creating a nationwide network to provide free or low-cost on-the-road access to commercial exercise facilities and those operated by the Department of Veterans Affairs (VA). The financial sustainability of trucker health requires creation of health savings account plans to incentivize healthy behaviors guided by population-based modeling and simulations.[10] Modeling should consider heterogeneity among populations of truckers: working conditions, the effects of government regulation, compensation practices, time away from home, and the impact of purchased out-of-pocket versus employer-paid insurance costs are markedly different between employed drivers and independent contractor owner-operators and between local delivery and long-distance over-the-road truckers.[11]

These variable features of trucking jobs serve as structural determinants of health that can be modified through deliberate design and regulation. Because improving trucker health involves many related actions and processes, the effort would benefit from integration through the tools of implementation science. VA clinicians have helped develop implementation science as a discipline to capture, codify, and create a policy framework for systematic adoption of successful behaviors and practices.[12]

Veteran truckers include individuals fully eligible for and dependent on VA health care and others without eligibility or who opt for non-VA care. All veteran truckers should be fully eligible for the population health and health savings account actions just noted and should be invited to engage in the VA's MOVE! and Whole Health programs (described subsequently).

EDUCATION AND ADVOCACY

Although metabolic risk is prevalent among truckers, it is also highly significant that about one third of the truckers involved in the studies cited here are not obese and are metabolically healthy.[2,3] These healthy veteran truckers are a critically important resource because they have learned how to incorporate into their jobs prudent diet options, adaptable on-the-road physical activity, relaxation techniques, and healthy sleep habits. They have the maturity, experience, and peer credibility to design, lead, and advocate for metabolic risk mitigation educational programs by serving on the veteran advisory panels that shape and assess such efforts in VA health facilities.[13] In addition, they should be engaged by the Task Force Movement partners—veteran service organizations, industry groups, and unions—who operate trucker apprenticeships to ensure that their CDL candidates gain robust health risk mitigation skills.[1]

Two existing VA programs have great potential for improving trucker health. The MOVE! program promotes healthy diet choices, weight reduction, and improved physical activity.[14] It gives veterans the ability to self-monitor their physical activity with Web-enabled Fitbit or Garmin monitors that can share data with providers to help motivate and sustain effort. The Whole Health program aims to provide a veteran-centered holistic framework for self-awareness and wellness, placing veterans at the center of care decisions and making use of in-person and Web-based tools that support mindfulness, relaxation techniques, and complementary or alternative therapy.[15] The White House task force recognizes the value of the whole health concept.[1] Truckers should receive no-cost remote access to telehealth and mobile telephone or video connectivity to support their engagement in MOVE! and Whole Health from any location.

The data collection period for the cited report of premature trucker mortality was 1985 to 2000.[4] New baselines and prospective monitoring are imperative if we are to engage in thoughtful implementation of new policies. We need to know the current health status of populations of over-the-road versus local delivery truckers and employed versus independent truckers to measure the effects of targeted actions over time. Aggregate data from CDL health assessments should be used to guide future actions. Task Force Movement should provide annual updates on the state of trucker health with a sharpened focus on measurable risk reduction outcomes.

Is it beyond our capability to change the future of metabolic syndrome risk factors, illness, and mortality among veteran truckers, all truckers, and all individuals? We think not, given the success of the United States' intentional public health efforts to decrease smoking in recent years and of the VA in its hepatitis C eradication effort. The veterans who will add to the trucker workforce are already experienced in applying the common military skill of risk mitigation to a new situation. It is clear that solving our supply chain and metabolic syndrome crises would benefit from convergence of our thinking and actions on both problems. Clinicians and leaders can and must ensure that the new truckers being recruited to improve our supply chain will be afforded strong protection from the adverse effects of the metabolic syndrome. AJPH

CORRESPONDENCE

Correspondence should be sent to Michael A. Dunn, MD, VA Northern Indiana Health Care System, 2121 Lake Ave, Fort Wayne, IN 46805 (e-mail: michael.dunn6@va.gov). Reprints can be ordered at http://www.ajph.org by clicking the "Reprints" link.

PUBLICATION INFORMATION

Full Citation: Dunn MA, Tapper EB, Rogal SS. Veteran truckers, the supply chain, and the metabolic syndrome: a convergence of crises. *Am J Public Health*. 2023;113(7):742–744.

Acceptance Date: April 15, 2023.

DOI: https://doi.org/10.2105/AJPH.2023.307321

CONTRIBUTORS

M. A. Dunn developed the concept and prepared the initial draft of the editorial. E. B. Tapper and S. S. Rogal provided important additional input to and revisions of the editorial.

ACKNOWLEDGMENTS

Michael A. Dunn receives support from the US Army Former Senior Strategic Leaders Conference. Elliot B. Tapper is supported by National Institutes of Health (NIH) grant U01DK130113. Shari S. Rogal is supported by NIH grant K23DA048182.

Note. The content is solely the responsibility of the authors and does not necessarily represent the official views of the NIH.

CONFLICTS OF INTEREST

There are no potential or actual conflicts of interest to disclose.

REFERENCES

1. White House. Task Force Movement partner convening conference. Available at: http://www.taskforcemovement.org. Accessed March 1, 2023.
2. Hege A, Lemke MK, Apostolopoulos Y, et al. Occupational health disparities among US long-haul truck drivers: the influence of work organization and sleep on cardiovascular and metabolic disease risk. *PLoS One*. 2018;13(11):e0207322. https://doi.org/10.1371/journal.pone.0207322
3. Bachmann LH, Lichtenstein B, St Lawrence JS, et al. Health risks of American long-distance truckers: results from a multisite assessment. *J Occup Environ Med*. 2018;60(7):e349–e355. https://doi.org/10.1097/JOM.0000000000001319
4. Laden F, Hart JE, Smith TJ, et al. Cause-specific mortality in the unionized US trucking industry. *Environ Health Perspect*. 2007;115(8):1192–1196. https://doi.org/10.1289/ehp.10027
5. *Risk Management: Department of the Army Pamphlet 385-30*. Washington, DC: US Department of the Army; 2014.
6. Federal Motor Carrier Safety Administration. Medical requirements for drivers. Available at: https://fmcsa.dot.gov/regulations/medical. Accessed March 1, 2023.
7. Mesinovic J, McMillan LB, Shore-Lorenti C, et al. Metabolic syndrome and its associations with components of sarcopenia in overweight and obese older adults. *J Clin Med*. 2019;8(2):145. https://doi.org/10.3390/jcm8020145
8. Vilar-Gomez E, Chalasani N. Non-invasive assessment of non-alcoholic fatty liver disease: clinical prediction rules and blood-based biomarkers. *J Hepatol*. 2018;68(2):305–315. https://doi.org/10.1016/j.jhep.2017.11.013
9. Johnson A, Cooper GF, Visweswaran S. Patient-specific modeling with personalized decision paths. *AMIA Annu Symp Proc*. 2021;2020:602–611.
10. Maglio PP, Sepulveda M-J, Mabry PL. Mainstreaming modeling and simulation to accelerate public health innovation. *Am J Public Health*. 2014;104(7):1181–1186. https://doi.org/10.2105/AJPH.2014.301873
11. Belzer MH. *Sweatshops on Wheels: Winners and Losers in Trucking Deregulation*. New York, NY: Oxford University Press; 2000.
12. Rogal SS, Powell BJ, Chinman M, et al. Moving toward impact: an introduction to implementation science for gastroenterologists and hepatologists. *Gastroenterology*. 2020;159(6):2007–2012. https://doi.org/10.1053/j.gastro.2020.07.063
13. Nearing KA, Adams HM, Alsphaugh J, et al. Engaging the wisdom of older veterans to enhance VA healthcare, research, and services. *J Gen Intern Med*. 2022;37(suppl 1):22–32. https://doi.org/10.1007/s11606-021-07076-x
14. Robinson KM, VanderWeg M, Laroche HH, et al. Obesity treatment initiation, retention, and outcomes in the Veterans Affairs MOVE! program among rural and urban veterans. *Obes Sci Pract*. 2022;8(6):784–793. https://doi.org/10.1002/osp4.622
15. Kligler B. Whole Health in the Veterans Health Administration. *Glob Adv Health Med*. 2022;11:2164957X221077214. https://doi.org/10.1177/2164957X221077214

Police Drug Seizures Cannot Solve the Problem of Toxic Drug Supply in North America

Paul Dietze, PhD

ABOUT THE AUTHOR

Paul Dietze is with the National Drug Research Institute, Melbourne Office, Curtin University, and the Burnet Institute, Melbourne, Victoria, Australia.

See also Stahler et al., p. 747, and Ray et al., p. 750.

In this issue of *AJPH*, Ray et al. (p. 750) present important findings on the relationships between local area indicators of drug market activity, focusing on the potential unintended consequences of local area drug law enforcement. Finding impacts of seizures on overdoses in subsequent days within local areas highlights the potential for unintended consequences of law enforcement activities on indicators of public health such as overdose.

The unintended consequences of law enforcement activities around drug markets and their impacts on people who use drugs have long been documented in a range of studies.[1,2] This ecological analysis by Ray et al. adds to this literature with an interesting hypothesis around a local area relationship between drug market supply and the tolerance of people who use drugs, long known as a risk factor for opioid overdose (e.g., Dietze et al.[3]). Ray et al. postulate two mechanisms by which market disruption and the removal of supply could impact tolerance—people who consume drugs may shift supply sources and obtain drugs of unknown quality that they cannot tolerate or they may reduce their use, leading to a reduction in tolerance. They indicate that they do not set out to specifically test these hypotheses, and the limitations of their cross-sectional ecological design precludes such hypothesis testing.

Indeed, the ready availability of high-potency opioids and stimulants in US drug markets[4] potentially undermines this argument because it is not clear whether the seizures in the study by Ray et al. actually disrupted drug supply or changed drug prices or the quality of available drugs. Previous work on the heroin market in Sydney, Australia, suggests that seizures have little impact on purity or availability in conditions where heroin was readily available,[5] often termed the heroin "glut" (a period of sustained ready availability of cheap, high-quality heroin),[6] and this may also apply to current drug markets in Indiana.

There are other potential explanatory mechanisms that may underpin the findings of Ray et al. Previous work has established that local area market disruption can lead to riskier patterns of use such as rushed injection or seeking out more deeply hidden places to use drugs.[7] These direct impacts observed in relation to street-based drug law enforcement may exacerbate the risks of overdose—for example, more deeply hidden spaces may limit the availability of response.[7] Alternatively, displacement to different places of drug use may also impact tolerance.[3] A fine-grained analysis of the locations of the overdoses in the study by Ray et al. could test whether displacement to riskier locations occurred in response to the seizures in their study. Complimentary studies with people who use drugs in the local areas could also help unpack the explanatory mechanisms of their findings. Furthermore, police presence and operations in drug markets antecedent to seizures may also produce displacement effects, and, so, cataloguing and studying police operations may help unpack the causal paths.

The relationship between drug law enforcement and public health is typically fraught. Performance indicators around street-level drug law enforcement are rarely specified beyond simple metrics such as arrests and seizures, which may not impact drug use and harms such as overdose. Nevertheless, drug supply is fundamentally important to illicit drug-related harms. The Australian heroin "drought," which occurred after the "glut,"[6] shows how a major interruption to supply can reduce key indicators of drug harms such as overdose.[6] However, although law enforcement operations are cited as one possible cause of the Australian heroin drought,[8] these claims are contested,[9] and there is currently no indication of any abatement of the toxic illicit drug supply in North America.

In the face of the North American overdose crisis, new approaches and policies around drugs are being trialed that involve partnerships between law enforcement and public health (e.g., Formica et al.[10]). Although there are serious concerns with some elements of these approaches,[11] and peer-led models may prove superior in the long run,[12] a dialogue between law enforcement and public health on their approach to drug law enforcement in the context of the overdose crisis is at least a step forward to the coordinated drug strategy required to reduce the devastating consequences of current practices in the United States. AJPH

CORRESPONDENCE

Correspondence should be sent to Professor Paul Dietze, National Drug Research Institute, Curtin University and Burnet Institute, 85 Commercial Rd, Melbourne, VIC 3004, Australia (e-mail: paul.dietze@burnet.edu.au). Reprints can be ordered at https://ajph.org by clicking the "Reprints" link.

PUBLICATION INFORMATION

Full Citation: Dietze P. Police drug seizures cannot solve the problem of toxic drug supply in North America. *Am J Public Health*. 2023;113(7):745–746.

Acceptance Date: April 21, 2023.

https://doi.org/10.2105/AJPH.2023.307328

CONFLICTS OF INTEREST

The author receives grant funding from the National Health and Medical Research Council and the Australian Government Department of Health.

REFERENCES

1. Aitken C, Moore D, Higgs P, Kelsall J, Kerger M. The impact of a police crackdown on a street drug scene: evidence from the street. *Int J Drug Policy*. 2002;13(3):193–202. https://doi.org/10.1016/S0955-3959(02)00075-0
2. Maher L, Dixon D. The cost of crackdowns: policing Cabramatta's heroin market. *Curr Issues Crim Justice*. 2001;13(1):5–22. https://doi.org/10.1080/10345329.2001.12036213
3. Dietze P, Jolley D, Fry C, Bammer G. Transient changes in behaviour lead to heroin overdose: results from a case-crossover study of non-fatal overdose. *Addiction*. 2005;100(5):636–642. https://doi.org/10.1111/j.1360-0443.2005.01051.x
4. Ciccarone D. The rise of illicit fentanyls, stimulants and the fourth wave of the opioid overdose crisis. *Curr Opin Psychiatry*. 2021;34(4):344–350. https://doi.org/10.1097/YCO.0000000000000717
5. Weatherburn D, Lind B. The impact of law enforcement activity on a heroin market. *Addiction*. 1997;92(5):557–569, discussion 611–553. https://doi.org/10.1111/j.1360-0443.1997.tb02913.x
6. Dietze P, Fitzgerald J. Interpreting changes in heroin supply in Melbourne: droughts, gluts or cycles? *Drug Alcohol Rev*. 2002;21(3):295–303. https://doi.org/10.1080/0959523021000002778
7. Fitzgerald J, Hamilton M, Dietze P. Walking overdoses: a re-appraisal of non-fatal illicit drug overdoses. *Addict Res*. 2000;8(4):327–355. https://doi.org/10.3109/16066350009009519
8. Degenhardt L, Day C, Gilmour S, Hall W. The "lessons" of the Australian "heroin shortage." *Subst Abuse Treat Prev Policy*. 2006;1(1):11. https://doi.org/10.1186/1747-597X-1-11
9. Wood E, Stoltz JA, Li K, Montaner JS, Kerr T. Changes in Canadian heroin supply coinciding with the Australian heroin shortage. *Addiction*. 2006;101(5):689–695. https://doi.org/10.1111/j.1360-0443.2006.01385.x
10. Formica SW, Reilly B, Duska M, et al. The Massachusetts Department of Public Health Post Overdose Support Team initiative: a public health-centered co-response model for post-overdose outreach. *J Public Health Manag Pract*. 2022;28(suppl 6):S311–S319. https://doi.org/10.1097/PHH.0000000000001574
11. Tori ME, Cummins E, Beletsky L, et al. Warrant checking practices by post-overdose outreach programs in Massachusetts: a mixed-methods study. *Int J Drug Policy*. 2022;100:103483. https://doi.org/10.1016/j.drugpo.2021.103483
12. Ray B, McCarthy-Nickila J, Richardson N, Maahs J. Post-overdose follow-up in the community with peer recovery specialists: the Lake Superior Diversion and Substance Use Response Team. *Drug Alcohol Depend Rep*. 2023;6:100139. https://doi.org/10.1016/j.dadr.2023.100139

At the Crossroads in the Opioid Overdose Epidemic: Will Evidence-Based "Radical" but Rational Drug Policy Strategies Prevail?

Gerald J. Stahler, PhD, Jeremy Mennis, PhD, and Steven Belenko, PhD

ABOUT THE AUTHORS

Gerald J. Stahler and Jeremy Mennis are with the Department of Geography and Urban Studies, Temple University, Philadelphia, PA. Steven Belenko is with the Department of Criminal Justice, Temple University.

See also Dietze, p. 745, and Ray et al., p. 750.

The current opioid drug overdose epidemic shows little sign of abating as more than 100 000 Americans needlessly died of drug overdose in 2022.[1] US efforts to mitigate this health crisis have been insufficient, and we need to reexamine our current drug policy priorities, practices, and strategies to ensure that they are based on science and empirical evidence. Ray et al., in this issue of *AJPH* (p. 750), examined the effects of police drug seizures on overdose in Indianapolis, Indiana, and found a consistent pattern of increased drug overdoses. The authors' findings suggest three strategic public health priorities that we believe are needed to improve our nation's response to the current opioid overdose crisis: (1) prioritizing cross-system and interorganizational collaborations to improve the effectiveness of existing health care and social service resources, (2) expanding the use of innovative geospatial data and methods to improve contextual understanding of policy and program effects, and (3) prioritizing demand reduction by expanding current harm-reduction approaches and implementing promising new "radical" but rational evidence-based interventions to save lives.

IMPROVING INTERORGANIZATIONAL LINKS

Ray et al. advocate greater collaboration among law enforcement and social service agencies that serve people who use drugs to prevent overdoses following police drug seizures. Prioritizing increased interorganizational links and collaborations is essential not only between law enforcement and service organizations but also across the many institutions and health care and social service systems already involved in mitigating addiction. The effectiveness of existing service system resources in the health care, addiction treatment, mental health, and social services sectors can be far more effective through lowered barriers and increased coordination, collaboration, linkages, and integration with one another to better serve the multiplicity of needs of people struggling with addiction. The siloing of these systems of care and lack of integration limits access to treatment and other needed services, especially for people of color, who are disproportionately affected by structural barriers such as poverty, racism, and stigmatization.

Unfortunately, fostering and sustaining these collaborations to reduce overdose is difficult given the disparate missions and cultures of different systems and agencies. The field of implementation science provides theoretical frameworks, interventions, measures, and tools to improve the uptake and implementation of evidence-based practices across systems, such as local change teams, needs assessments, coaching and feedback, and data-driven decision-making.[2] A good example of this approach involves the National Institute on Drug Abuse's Justice Community Opioid Innovation Network (JCOIN) initiative. Because of the high prevalence of opioid use disorder among people under criminal justice supervision, this network's projects are using implementation science methods to guide the development and evaluation of interventions that facilitate and sustain linkages between criminal justice systems and treatment organizations to improve access to opioid use disorder services.[3]

USING INNOVATIVE GEOSPATIAL METHODS

Ray et al. also illustrate the significant contributions that geospatial analysis can make to understanding and addressing addiction. Geospatial data

AJPH July 2023, Vol 113, No. 7

capture key social and environmental determinants of health that relate to substance use, such as neighborhood disadvantage, segregation, and access to health care.[4] Novel mapping and geospatial statistical techniques, such as spatiotemporal clustering, use such data to reveal how environmental and biopsychosocial factors interact to influence substance use behaviors and treatment outcomes, both among individuals and across communities.[5] Interdisciplinary collaboration between public health researchers and geospatial scientists is key to advancing the effectiveness of drug policies, prevention, and intervention programs aimed at reducing overdose and other harms.

PROMISING RADICAL HARM-REDUCTION POLICIES

Although opioid overprescribing may have fueled the overdose crisis by increasing drug supply,[6] Ray et al. illustrate the limitations and complexities of relying on supply-side interventions targeting the illicit drug market. Consistent with previous research concerning local drug supply disruptions, the increased incidence of overdose in their study likely resulted from reduced tolerance among users who cannot easily access opioids, increased use of unfamiliar fentanyl-contaminated polydrug combinations, and seeking out unfamiliar drug sellers who provide drugs with unknown potency.[7]

Between 2014 and 2022, federal funding for supply reduction efforts (e.g., law enforcement and interdiction) comprised 52% of the federal drug control budget. We are encouraged that the fiscal year 2023 budget request for President Biden's administration's latest national drug control strategy devotes 57% to demand reduction. The strategy includes harm reduction as one of its seven major policy priorities, along with advancing racial equity in drug policy and expanding recovery support services (https://bit.ly/43H7U6u; https://bit.ly/3MW3nqS). Also, recent federal regulatory changes will increase access to buprenorphine and naloxone.

Unfortunately, even with massive efforts to link existing systems, expand prevention programs, and increase access to evidence-based opioid use disorder treatment, there will still be people who use drugs who do not have an opioid use disorder but still use opioids, people with opioid use disorder who are either not yet ready to engage in treatment or will never seek treatment, and many for whom treatment has been either effective or ineffective who return to drug use. The increasingly lethal illicit street drug supply, in which fentanyl, xylazine, and other dangerous adulterants predominate, places these people at great risk for overdose.

You cannot treat the dead. It is for groups of high-risk people that two additional so-called "radical" but promising evidence-based harm-reduction interventions are needed to save lives: overdose prevention sites and safe supply policies.

Research evidence suggests that overdose prevention sites (i.e., safe injection sites), where people who use drugs inject under medical supervision, are effective in reducing overdose deaths and serve as a low barrier gateway to treatment and other services without increasing opioid use or crime.[8,9] More than 160 sites have been implemented in Europe, Canada, and Australia, and two sites are currently operating in New York City, with others planned in Rhode Island and Philadelphia, Pennsylvania.[9] Rigorous evaluations informed by implementation science should be undertaken to assess the implementation and effectiveness of these sites, including how best to facilitate low barrier linkages to treatment and other services.

Serious consideration should also be given to modifying current prescribing regulations to examine safe supply interventions, such as heroin-assisted treatment, in which pharmaceutical grade opioids (e.g., hydromorphone and diacetylmorphine) are prescribed to divert people who use drugs to safer alternatives and away from the unregulated illicit drug market, where there is high risk for overdose.[10] One recent systematic review found substantial evidence of heroin-assisted treatment effectiveness in increased treatment retention and reduced illegal drug use compared with methadone maintenance treatment.[11]

As Ray et al. illustrate, addressing the opioid overdose crisis strictly through supply-side interventions is unlikely to be successful, as the United States' long history of prohibitionist drug control policies have shown.[6] Considering the current lethality of the opioid crisis, greater interorganizational linkages and collaborations are needed among treatment, health care, social services, criminal justice, and harm-reduction organizations to reduce treatment barriers and increase access to needed services. Harm-reduction interventions should be scaled up for those most at risk for overdose, including overdose prevention sites and safe supply prescribing policies, and rigorously evaluated with both traditional research and innovative geospatial and implementation science methodologies. Our systems of care need to provide equitable, nonstigmatizing, and respectful services for all individuals who currently use drugs regardless of their stage in the recovery continuum.[12] AJPH

CORRESPONDENCE

Correspondence should be sent to Gerald Stahler, PhD, Department of Geography and Urban Studies, 343 Gladfelter Hall, 1115 Pollett Walk, Temple University (025-27), Philadelphia, PA 19122 (e-mail: jstahler@temple.edu). Reprints can be ordered at http://www.ajph.org by clicking the "Reprints" link.

PUBLICATION INFORMATION

Full Citation: Stahler GJ, Mennis J, Belenko S. At the crossroads in the opioid overdose epidemic: will evidence-based "radical" but rational drug policy strategies prevail? *Am J Public Health*. 2023; 113(7):747–749.

Acceptance Date: April 15, 2023.

DOI: https://doi.org/10.2105/AJPH.2023.307320

CONTRIBUTORS

G. J. Stahler conceptualized the editorial and outlined the first draft. All authors drafted and edited the editorial.

ACKNOWLEDGMENTS

G. J. Stahler and S. Belenko were supported by the National Institutes of Health (NIH), Helping to End Addiction Long-Term Initiative through the National Institute on Drug Abuse (NIDA), Justice Community Opioid Innovation Network (award number 1U01DA050442-01; Rosemarie Martin, principal investigator).

We would like to thank Jose Benitez and Silvana Mazzella for their insights over many years regarding harm reduction.

Note. The funders had no role in the preparation of this editorial. The content is solely the responsibility of the authors and does not necessarily represent the official views of the NIH or NIDA.

CONFLICTS OF INTEREST

G. J. Stahler serves as an unpaid member of the board of directors of Prevention Point Philadelphia, a nonprofit harm-reduction organization, , and as an unpaid member of a committee of the board of directors of Gaudenzia, Inc, a nonprofit drug treatment organization. The other authors have no conflicts of interest to declare.

REFERENCES

1. Ahmad FB, Cisewski JA, Rossen LM, Sutton P. Provisional drug overdose death counts. February 15, 2023. Available at: https://www.cdc.gov/nchs/nvss/vsrr/drug-overdose-data.htm. Accessed January 28, 2023.
2. Powell BJ, Waltz TJ, Chinman MJ, et al. A refined compilation of implementation strategies: results from the Expert Recommendations for Implementing Change (ERIC) project. *Implement Sci.* 2015;10:21. https://doi.org/10.1186/s13012-015-0209-1
3. Ducharme LJ, Wiley TRA, Mulford CF, Su ZI, Zur JB. Engaging the justice system to address the opioid crisis: the Justice Community Opioid Innovation Network (JCOIN). *J Subst Abuse Treat.* 2021;128:108307. https://doi.org/10.1016/j.jsat.2021.108307
4. Mennis J, Stahler GJ, Mason MJ. Risky substance use environments and addiction: a new frontier for environmental justice research. *Int J Environ Res Public Health.* 2016;13(6):607. https://doi.org/10.3390/ijerph13060607
5. Stahler GJ, Mennis J. Geospatial technology and the "exposome": new perspectives on addiction. *Am J Public Health.* 2013;103(8):1354–1356. https://doi.org/10.2105/AJPH.2013.301306
6. Gottschalk M. The opioid crisis: the war on drugs is over. Long live the war on drugs. *Annu Rev Criminol.* 2023;6:363–398. https://doi.org/10.1146/annurev-criminol-030421-040140
7. Beletsky L, Davis CS. Today's fentanyl crisis: prohibition's iron law, revisited. *Int J Drug Policy.* 2017;46:156–159. https://doi.org/10.1016/j.drugpo.2017.05.050
8. Naeem AH, Davis CS, Samuels EA. The importance of federal action supporting overdose-prevention centers. *N Engl J Med.* 2022;386(21):1965–1967. https://doi.org/10.1056/NEJMp2119764
9. Stahler GJ. *Safe Injection Sites as a Public Health Response to the Opioid Crisis: Research Evidence and Policy Recommendations.* Philadelphia, PA: Temple University Public Policy Lab; 2022. Public Policy Brief No. 16. Available at: https://drive.google.com/file/d/1LbHUQdKgqhn2TXe7LkwHFWGEXtKVyg1M/view. Accessed April 18, 2023.
10. McNeil R, Fleming T, Mayer S, et al. Implementation of safe supply alternatives during intersecting COVID-19 and overdose health emergencies in British Columbia, Canada, 2021. *Am J Public Health.* 2022;112(suppl 2):S151–S158. https://doi.org/10.2105/AJPH.2021.306692
11. McNair R, Monaghan M, Montgomery P. Heroin assisted treatment for key health outcomes in people with chronic heroin addictions: a context-focused systematic review. *Drug Alcohol Depend.* [In press]. https://doi.org/10.1016/j.drugalcdep.2023.109869
12. Volkow ND. Drug overdose deaths in 2020 were horrifying. Radical change is needed to address the drug crisis. National Institute on Drug Abuse. August 31, 2021. Available at: https://nida.nih.gov/about-nida/noras-blog/2021/08/drug-overdose-deaths-in-2020-were-horrifying-radical-change-needed-to-address-drug-crisis. Accessed March 26, 2023.

Spatiotemporal Analysis Exploring the Effect of Law Enforcement Drug Market Disruptions on Overdose, Indianapolis, Indiana, 2020–2021

Bradley Ray, PhD, Steven J. Korzeniewski, PhD, George Mohler, PhD, Jennifer J. Carroll, PhD, MPH, Brandon del Pozo, PhD, Grant Victor, PhD, Philip Huynh, MPH, and Bethany J. Hedden, MSW

See also Dietze, p. 745, and Stahler et al., p. 747.

Objectives. To test the hypothesis that law enforcement efforts to disrupt local drug markets by seizing opioids or stimulants are associated with increased spatiotemporal clustering of overdose events in the surrounding geographic area.

Methods. We performed a retrospective (January 1, 2020 to December 31, 2021), population-based cohort study using administrative data from Marion County, Indiana. We compared frequency and characteristics of drug (i.e., opioids and stimulants) seizures with changes in fatal overdose, emergency medical services nonfatal overdose calls for service, and naloxone administration in the geographic area and time following the seizures.

Results. Within 7, 14, and 21 days, opioid-related law enforcement drug seizures were significantly associated with increased spatiotemporal clustering of overdoses within radii of 100, 250, and 500 meters. For example, the observed number of fatal overdoses was two-fold higher than expected under the null distribution within 7 days and 500 meters following opioid-related seizures. To a lesser extent, stimulant-related drug seizures were associated with increased spatiotemporal clustering overdose.

Conclusions. Supply-side enforcement interventions and drug policies should be further explored to determine whether they exacerbate an ongoing overdose epidemic and negatively affect the nation's life expectancy. (*Am J Public Health*. 2023;113(7):750–758. https://doi.org/10.2105/AJPH.2023.307291)

AJPH July 2023, Vol 113, No. 7

The overdose epidemic has accounted for nearly 1 million lives lost in the United States in the past 2 decades.[1] Although the majority of overdose deaths are opioid related, the type of opioid involved and corresponding mortality rates vary over time, with fentanyl presently driving the fatality count in opioid- and stimulant-involved overdose deaths alike.[2,3] Emergency medical services (EMS) are typically deployed in response to overdose and poisoning calls for service, and EMS administer naloxone (an opioid antagonist) when indicated to reverse respiratory depression caused by opioids. Although there are substantial geographic and policy differences in who administers naloxone and under what circumstnaces,[4] the number of EMS naloxone administrations per capita are increasingly used for public health surveillance purposes[5] and to guide resource allocation.[6] However, the search continues to identify factors that reliably precede overdoses to trigger and inform targeted prevention efforts.[7–9] We explored law enforcement drug market disruptions as a potential factor.

People can develop a tolerance for opioids, although overdose occurs when dosage exceeds tolerance to the point of respiratory failure. Unknown opioid tolerance at relapse is a documented overdose risk factor among the recently incarcerated[10,11] and those discharged from residential treatment and withdrawal management settings.[12,13] Reductions in tolerance can occur after any involuntary disruption of an individual's opioid supply, and accidentally ingesting a dose beyond one's tolerance can be fatal. This mechanism accounts for the second wave of the overdose epidemic, when consumers shifted from pharmaceutical opioids to heroin. Heroin is a much less consistent and predictable product, increasing the dangers that come of unknown tolerance, especially overdose risk.[2,14]

This same mechanism has been documented as occurring in the illicit drug market following disruptions from an arrested supplier and consumers contending with new and potentially unfamiliar products.[15,16] The impact of these drug market disruptions may be particularly salient for people who use opioids, who can experience painful withdrawal symptoms and diminished biological tolerance even after short periods of abstinence.[13] There is also a risk for people who knowingly use stimulants but are opioid naïve and, thus, have lower opioid tolerance; they might seek a new supplier following a drug market disruption and then overdose from fentanyl-contaminated stimulants.[3]

We tested the hypothesis that law enforcement efforts to disrupt local drug markets through routine supply-side interdictions—as measured by police seizures of opioid- and stimulant-related substances—are associated with increased spatiotemporal clustering of fatal and nonfatal overdoses, as well as increases in EMS naloxone administration, in the area surrounding the seizure. Although the analytical methods we employed cannot establish causality, we hypothesized that the causal mechanism for an association lies in the disruption of a person's ability to obtain a substance they can accurately dose; this is because that supply has become unavailable, resulting in their transition to an alternate supply with no knowledge of its potency or their ensuing tolerance.[11,13,15] Given the potential for withdrawal and overdose because of unknown tolerance among opioid users, we hypothesized an association with EMS naloxone administration following opioid-related seizures. But with the potential for unintentional opioid consumption among stimulant users, we also explored naloxone administration associated with stimulant-related seizures.

METHODS

We performed a retrospective, 2-year, population-based study by using administrative data from Marion County, Indiana. Marion County is the largest county in the state, with a population of nearly 1 million, and is home to Indianapolis, the state capital and 15th largest city in the nation.[17] We selected Marion County because it accounts for a quarter of Indiana's overdose deaths, with a mortality rate higher than the national average, and because of the availability of point-level event information across multiple data sources that are required to test our spatiotemporal hypothesis. The 3 sources of data collected between January 1, 2020, and December 31, 2021, and used in this study included (1) property room drug seizure data from the Indianapolis Metropolitan Police Department, (2) fatal overdose data from the Marion County Coroner's Office, and (3) nonfatal overdose calls for service and naloxone administration data from the Indianapolis Emergency Medical Services.

We conducted our analyses using R version 4.2.0 (RStudio, Boston, MA).

Drug Interdiction

Information on drug seizures included the location (street address), time, date, and physical description of the substance (based largely on law enforcement observation and discernment of the substances). We removed all incidents (which are not mutually exclusive) in which a drug seizure was not disruptive (e.g., a police-controlled purchase as part of an investigation, a found substance); that took place in a geographical area not in the community (e.g., an airport or hospital, police facilities where materials are identified); or that did not meet substance criteria (i.e., seizures of substances other than opioids or stimulants or consisting of only drug paraphernalia). We removed drug seizures with unknown or missing drug incident data and then subclassified seizures as opioid related (e.g., fentanyl, heroin, morphine, prescription opioids) or stimulant related (e.g., amphetamines, cocaine, methamphetamines) based on the reported descriptions.

Per administrative property room data, each confiscated item is considered a unique event; therefore, 1 incident could have multiple items, and we included each item as an event in this study. Thus, events do not refer to the number of law enforcement interdiction events, but the number of times opioids or stimulants were logged across all interdiction events. Although information on precise quantity is limited because of the lack of confirmatory toxicological results on the seized samples, we normalized information to metric grams and used Indiana criminal codes to determine that 10.4% of all drug seizures were considered large

(Table A, available as a supplement to the online version of this article at http://www.ajph.org).

Fatal and Nonfatal Overdoses

We looked at 3 overdose outcomes. We identified fatal overdoses using the death certificate and toxicology results for all accidental drug overdose events (code X40-X44 of *International Classification of Diseases, 10th Revision* [Geneva, Switzerland: World Health Organization; 1992]) from coroner records. Toxicology data provided information about substances detected using thresholds set by the testing agency, and we determined location from the place of injury. However, we examined fatal overdoses without subclassification by underlying substance because most were polydrug overdoses. We defined nonfatal overdoses as any event in which naloxone was administered and a chief complaint or mechanism of injury was recorded as overdose or poisoning, and we looked separately at the naloxone administration event. Although other sources provide nonfatal overdose data (e.g., emergency departments), we chose EMS events based on previous research[18] and the ability to measure their spatiotemporal proximity to seizures, removing events that occurred in a hospital setting.

Statistical Analyses

In our primary analysis, we first used the Knox test statistic (κ) to identify excess space–time clustering between police seizures of opioid- and stimulant-related drugs and drug overdose events occurring in the surrounding area over a specific interval of time. To further explore potential time order of associations, we then tested for differences in space–time clustering of overdose events before versus after police drug seizures ($\Delta\kappa$).

Magnitudes of association. Informed by earlier studies,[19,20] we calculated the 2-sample Knox test statistic (κ) to identify excess space–time clustering between police drug seizures (i.e., opioid related and stimulant related) and overdose (i.e., fatal overdose, nonfatal overdose, and naloxone administration), where κ consists of the count of overdose events within τ days and a radius of δ meters of drug seizures:

$$(1)\quad \kappa = \sum_{(i,j)} 1\{|\,(|\,x_i^s - x_j^o\,|)\,| < \delta,\ |\,t_i^s - t_j^o\,| < \tau\}.$$

In equation 1, x_i^s (t_i^s) is the location (time) of drug seizure i, x_j^o (t_j^o) is the location (time) of overdose event j, and 1 is the indicator function. To determine excess clustering of overdose events, we compared the Knox statistic with a null hypothesis in which the 2 processes are independent, with the null distribution constructed by randomly shuffling event times t_i^s of the drug seizures while keeping the locations and event times of the overdoses fixed. We used 200 realizations of reshuffled event times to quantify uncertainty in the null distribution of κ to disentangle the time ordering of drug seizures and overdose events with the following form, where the count of overdoses within a radius of δ meters and τ days before a seizure was subtracted from the count of overdoses within a radius of δ meters and τ days after a seizure:

$$(2)\quad \Delta\kappa = \sum_{(i,j)} 1\{\|\,x_i^s - x_j^o\,\| < \delta, 0 < t_j^o - t_i^s < \tau\} - \sum_{(i,j)} 1\{\|\,x_i^s - x_j^o\,\| < \delta, -\tau < t_j^o - t_i^s < 0\},$$

Based on previous research,[21] we examined radii of 100, 250, and 500 meters at durations of 7, 14, and 21 days, respectively, and given the total number of seizure events, we report our results in all figures, supplemental tables, and text as per 100 seizure events.

Pre–post differences. Because overdose events can occur before and after drug seizures, we used a pre–post design to establish time order. First, we estimated a 95% confidence interval (CI) for the expected difference in overdose events under a null distribution (i.e., no association between police seizure and overdose events) of pre–post test differences (i.e., $\Delta\kappa$, which can be positive or negative, with a positive value of $\Delta\kappa$ indicating more overdose events cluster after drug seizures) by resampling. We then calculated observed pre–post test differences in event rates. Observed numbers of drug overdose events per 100 police drug seizures (κ) and pre–post test differences ($\Delta\kappa$) that lie outside the 95% CIs estimated under the null hypothesis of no association are statistically significant.

RESULTS

Figure 1 describes how we arrived at the final sample of opioid- and stimulant-related drug seizures, and Figure 2 displays their association with overdose events (fatal and combined nonfatal events) in 6-month increments over the 24-month study period (Figure A [available as a supplement to the online version of this article at http://www.ajph.org] animates the daily patterns). There were 2110 opioid-related and 3039 stimulant-related drug seizures during the 24-month study period, representing an average of 7.0 drug seizures per day (range = 0–22). The mean for opioids and stimulants, respectively, was 2.9 and 4.2 drug seizures per day. Death data showed 1171 fatal overdoses, and EMS data showed 12 590 nonfatal overdoses, of which 51.0%

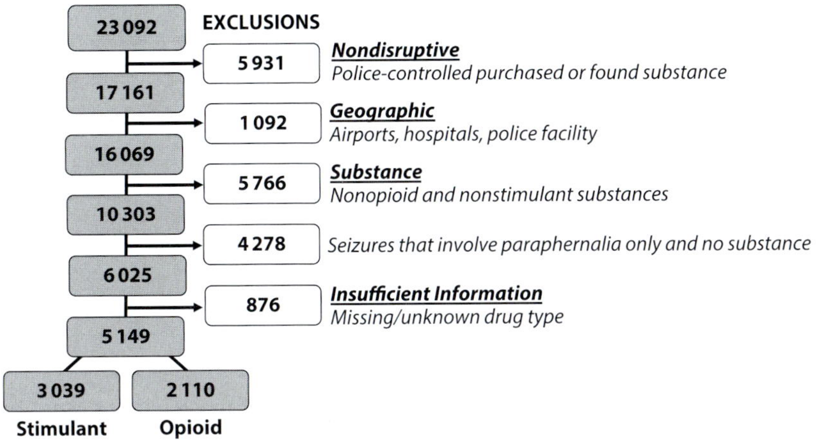

FIGURE 1— Case Determination of Drug Seizure Events From Property Room Data to Determine Final Sample: Marion County, IN, 2020–2021

Note. Records ranged from January 1, 2020, to December 31, 2021, and included 23 092 seizure events. Nondisruptive seizures included those coded as found, stolen, or nonevidentiary, whereas geographic removals included 98 events at an airport or hospital and 944 events with the police district coded as the location. For substance exclusions, 84.1% of the 5766 substances that were not coded as opioids or stimulants were cannabis related. After these exclusion criteria, there were 14.5% (n = 876) events without complete information on the substance or location, resulting in a final sample of 5149. Seizure events were not mutually exclusive because 244 cases were both opioid and stimulant related.

(n = 6419) included naloxone administration. These data represent an average of 1.6 fatal overdoses per day (range = 0–7), 17.2 nonfatal overdoses per day (range = 4–35), and 8.8 naloxone administrations per day (range = 0–21).

Magnitudes of Association

Police seizures described as opioids were significantly associated with spatiotemporal clustering of fatal overdoses, nonfatal overdoses, and naloxone administrations at all selected time and distance parameters used in the analysis (100 m at 7 days, 250 m at 14 days, 500 m at 21 days; Figure 3; Figure B [available as a supplement to the online version of this article at http://www.ajph.org] provides the full set of comparisons). For example, the expected number of fatal overdoses within 500 meters and 21 days of opioid-related drug seizures ranged from 18.0 to 22.7 per 100 drug seizures, so the observed rate of 23.6 was higher than expected under the estimated null distribution. Stimulant-related drug seizures were also significantly associated with increased spatiotemporal clustering of overdose events but only at a distance of 100 meters within 7 days; the pattern of association was stronger for nonfatal overdoses.

Pre–Post Differences

Figure 4 shows the observed pre–post drug seizure differences in overdose events versus what was expected under the null distribution (Figure C [available as a supplement to the online version of this article at http://www.ajph.org] shows the same for all time and distance parameters used in the analysis). The difference in fatal overdoses and naloxone administrations before and after opioid-related seizures was significantly greater than expected under the null distribution. By contrast, only at a distance of 100 meters over 7 days were the observed pre–post test differences in nonfatal overdoses higher than expected under the null distribution.

There were fewer statistically different changes from the estimated null distribution following stimulant-related seizures. Only at 100 meters within 7 days was the observed pre–post test difference in fatal overdoses following stimulant-related seizures higher than expected under the estimated null distribution. Moreover, the observed pre–post test difference in nonfatal overdoses with stimulant-related drug seizures was lower than expected compared with the estimated null distribution only at 250 meters within 14 days.

DISCUSSION

Our population-based study provides evidence that police seizures of substances identified as opioids or stimulants are significantly associated with increased spatiotemporal clustering of overdose events in the immediate surrounding geographic area (radii of 100 m, 250 m, and 500 m) over 1-, 2-, and 3-week periods. Importantly, the difference in spatiotemporal clustering of all 3 overdose event rates before and after opioid-related seizures was higher than expected under the estimated null distribution across all radii and time intervals although this pattern of association was less consistent among stimulant-related seizures. This is consistent with our hypothesized mechanism because persons with opioid use disorder who lose their supply will experience both diminishing tolerance and withdrawal, whereby even the anticipation of painful symptoms may lead them to seek a new supply while discounting risks that stem from the differences in potency inherent in an

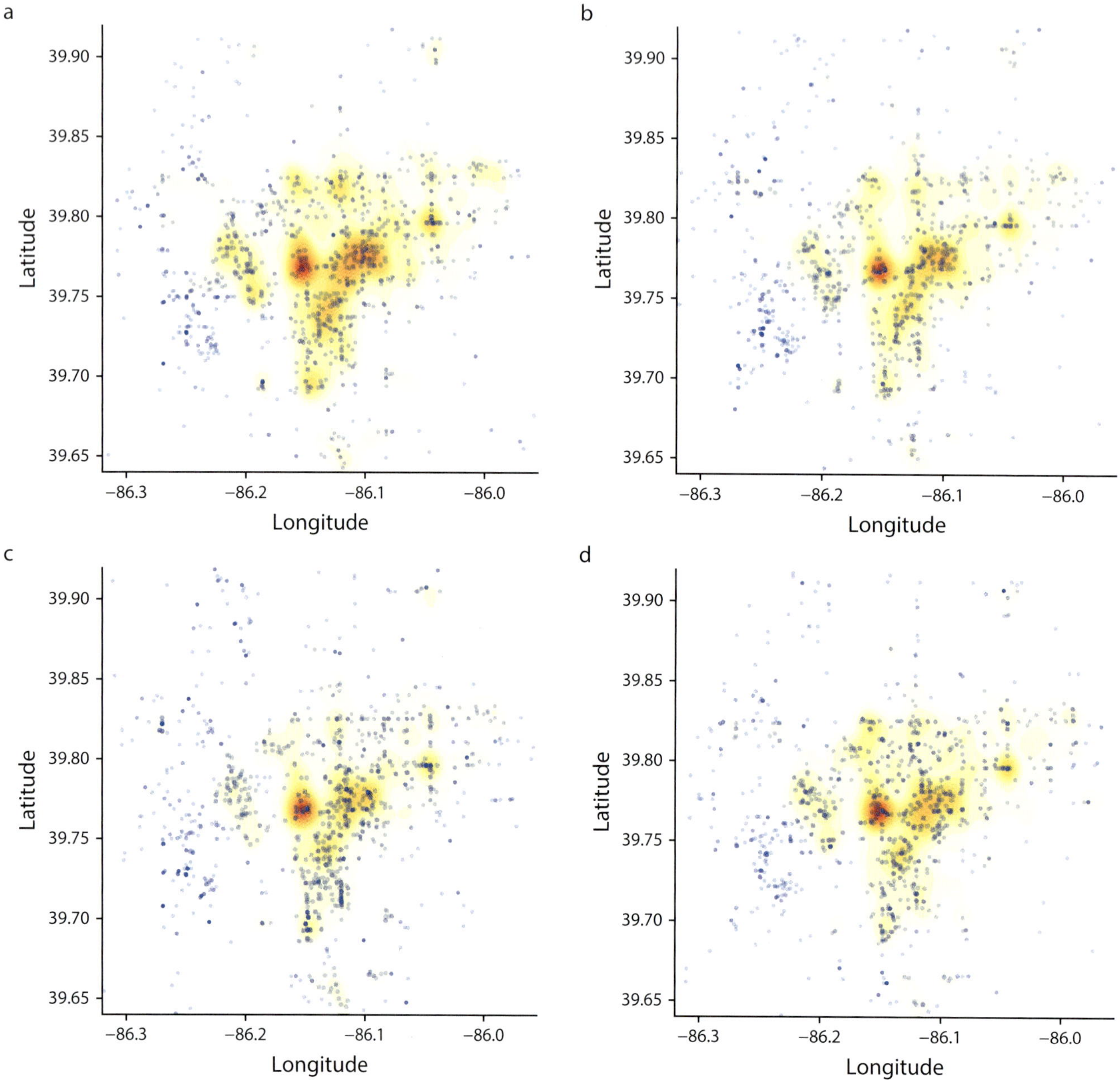

FIGURE 2— **Drug Seizures (Opioid-Related and Stimulant-Related) and Overdose (Fatal Overdose, Nonfatal Overdose, and Naloxone Administration) Events Over 6-Month Increments (a) Jan 1–Jun 30, 2020, (b) Jul 1–Dec 31, 2020, (c) Jan 1–Jun 30, 2021, and (d) Jul 1–Dec 31, 2021: Indianapolis, IN**

Note. Drug seizures include both opioid- and stimulant-related events; overdose events include both fatal and nonfatal, which include naloxone administrations.

illicit opioid market; this results in unknown tolerance, uncertainty about a safe dose, and increased overdose risk.

We were unable to assert a causal relationship between law enforcement drug market disruptions and overdose, and our study was not designed to, but our results are consistent with other evidence of this association.[18,19,22–24] Moreover, federal agencies already recognize the harms that emerge from these disruptions; for example, the Centers for Disease Control and Prevention developed the Opioid Rapid Response Program, an interagency effort designed to reduce overdose by rapidly increasing access to treatment of chronic pain and substance use disorder in the wake of enforcement actions against pain clinics and opioid prescribers.[25,26] Routine supply-side interdictions among police may merit similar efforts to prevent resulting overdose in the surrounding community—but with more frequent

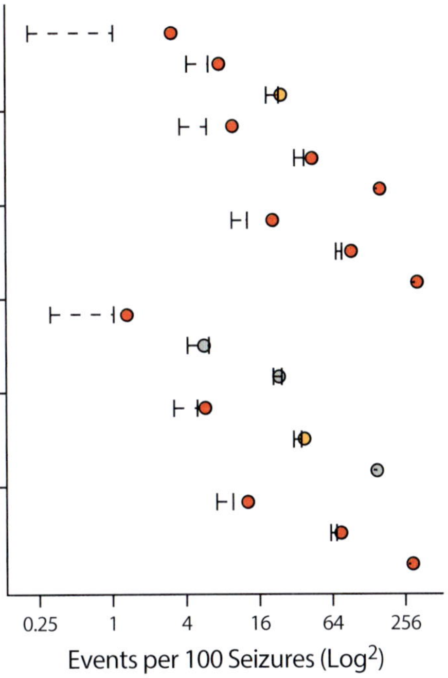

Seizure	Event	Distance (Time)	Observed K	Expected Null (95% CI)	FC	P
Opioid-Related Seizure	Fatal overdose	100 m (7 d)	3.0	0.6 (0.2, 1.0)	4.9	<.001
		250 m (14 d)	7.3	5.0 (4.0, 6.0)	1.4	<.001
		500 m (21 d)	23.6	20.4 (18.0, 22.7)	1.2	.009
	Nonfatal overdose	100 m (7 d)	9.5	4.6 (3.5, 5.8)	2.1	<.001
		250 m (14 d)	43.5	33.9 (30.7, 36.9)	1.3	<.001
		500 m (21 d)	154.6	142.2 (136.9, 147.7)	1.1	<.001
	Naloxone admin.	100 m (7 d)	20.1	10.9 (9.3, 12.5)	1.8	<.001
		250 m (14 d)	88.9	71.4 (67.3, 75.0)	1.2	<.001
		500 m (21 d)	317.3	296.6 (286.7, 305.4)	1.1	<.001
Stimulant-Related Seizure	Fatal overdose	100 m (7 d)	1.3	0.6 (0.3, 1.0)	2.3	<.001
		250 m (14 d)	5.4	5.1 (4.0, 6.0)	1.0	.641
		500 m (21 d)	22.8	21.9 (20.3, 23.8)	1.0	.325
	Nonfatal overdose	100 m (7 d)	5.6	3.9 (3.1, 4.8)	1.4	<.001
		250 m (14 d)	36.3	32.4 (29.9, 34.7)	1.1	.001
		500 m (21 d)	144.7	140.6 (135.8, 145.4)	1.0	.091
	Naloxone admin.	100 m (7 d)	12.4	8.2 (6.9, 9.4)	1.5	<.001
		250 m (14 d)	72.5	63.8 (60.2, 67.3)	1.1	<.001
		500 m (21 d)	286.1	273.2 (265.6, 279.0)	1.0	<.001

FIGURE 3— Spatiotemporal Associations Between Opioid-Related and Stimulant-Related Drug Seizures and Fatal Overdose, Nonfatal Overdose, and Naloxone Administration Events: Marion County, IN, 2020–2021

Note. admin = administration; CI = confidence interval; FC = fold change observed vs expected.

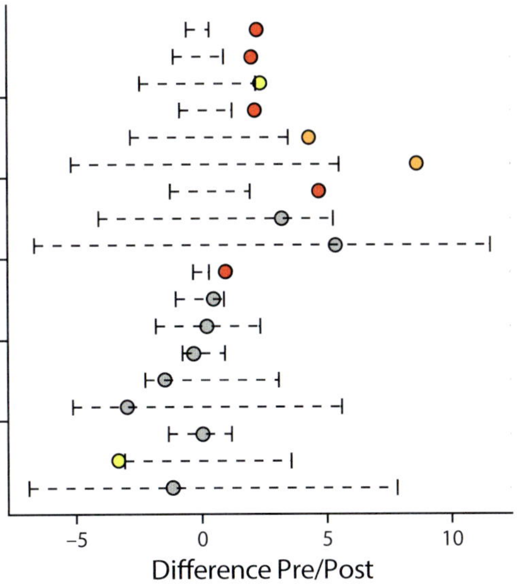

Exposure	Event	Distance (Time)	Observed Difference	Expected Null[a] (95% CI)	FC	P
Opioid-Related Exposure	Fatal overdose	100 m (7 d)	2.2	(−0.6, 0.3)	7.8	<.001
		250 m (14 d)	2.0	(−1.1, 0.9)	1.8	<.001
		500 m (21 d)	2.4	(−2.4, 2.2)	1.2	.049
	Naloxone admin.	100 m (7 d)	2.1	(−0.9, 1.2)	1.6	<.001
		250 m (14 d)	4.3	(−2.8, 3.5)	1.2	.01
		500 m (21 d)	8.6	(−5.2, 5.5)	1.1	.006
	Nonfatal overdose	100 m (7 d)	4.7	(−1.2, 1.9)	1.6	<.001
		250 m (14 d)	3.2	(−4.1, 5.3)	1.1	.297
		500 m (21 d)	5.4	(−6.6, 11.6)	1.0	.46
Stimulant-Related Exposure	Fatal overdose	100 m (7 d)	1.0	(−0.3, 0.3)	7.0	<.001
		250 m (14 d)	0.5	(−1.0, 0.9)	1.2	.281
		500 m (21 d)	0.2	(−1.8, 2.3)	1.0	.963
	Naloxone admin.	100 m (7 d)	−0.3	(−0.8, 0.9)	0.9	.31
		250 m (14 d)	−1.5	(−2.2, 3.1)	0.9	.208
		500 m (21 d)	−3.0	(−5.1, 5.6)	1.0	.207
	Nonfatal overdose	100 m (7 d)	0.0	(−1.3, 1.2)	1.0	.925
		250 m (14 d)	−3.3	(−3.1, 3.6)	0.9	.028
		500 m (21 d)	−1.2	(−6.9, 7.8)	1.0	.58

FIGURE 4— Observed vs Expected Pre–Post Differences in Spatiotemporal Associations Between Opioid-Related and Stimulant-Related Drug Seizures and Fatal Overdose, Nonfatal Overdose, and Naloxone Administration Events: Marion County, IN, 2020–2021

Note. admin = administration; CI = confidence interval; FC = fold change observed vs expected.
[a]The observed pre–post difference is compared to the 95% CI for the expected difference estimated under the null distribution.

need, given the prevailing volume of seizures.

Officers might also use the considerable discretion at their disposal when interacting with persons who use drugs, particularly in enforcing misdemeanors or nonviolent felonies that regulate drugs to reduce harms that might come from disrupting an individual's drug supply.[27] Additionally, our study suggests that information on drug seizures may provide a touchpoint that is further upstream than other postoverdose events, providing greater potential to mitigate harms. For example, although the role of law enforcement in overdose remains a topic of debate,[28] public safety partnerships could entail timely notice of interdiction events to agencies that provide overdose prevention services, outreach, and referral to care.[25]

Efforts to disrupt the illicit drug supply have historically incentivized potency to minimize volume (and therefore transportation risk) and maximize profit, bringing the United States from an overdose epidemic fueled by prescription medications to illicitly manufactured fentanyl.[29] As drug markets become less predictable and morbidity and mortality among people who use drugs increases, it is critical that communities not only create low barrier access to evidence-based treatment but also implement harm reduction strategies that directly address supply-side drivers of accidental overdose. Naloxone distribution, drug-checking, and overdose prevention sites are strategies first developed and implemented by people who use drugs that can be facilitated or enhanced by law enforcement cooperation through exceptions or "carve-outs" of drug criminalization to protect public health.[30,31] These practices provide people who use drugs with shelter from the harms of drug policy but fall short of reassessing and revising policies that might prevent these harms in the first place.[32,33]

Moreover, to explore whether policies or practices affect the association between seizures and overdose observed in this study, it is critically important to replicate our analysis in other jurisdictions that are more or less punitive to determine whether seizures are associated with overdose in jurisdictions where people have access to a wider range of overdose prevention practices. For example, Indiana's Good Samaritan Law (Indiana Code Title 16. Health § 16-42-27–2(g)-(h)) provides immunity from prosecution for drug possession provided the person administered naloxone and remained on the scene to cooperate with first responders. However, this law offers no protections for the overdose victim, which is uncommon for such laws and may contribute to decreased overdose calls for service in Indianapolis.[34] Additionally, although a legal framework for syringe service programs is in place, the unauthorized possession of syringes remains a felony crime in Indiana (Indiana Code Title 16. Health § 16-42-19-18) and may contribute to arrest following overdose calls for service,[35] likewise creating hesitancy to summon help.

Limitations

As with all observational studies, we cannot infer causality from the statistical associations. Although our use of the Knox test was novel and well suited to test our spatiotemporal hypothesis, it did not allow us to consider the influence of community-level factors that might affect results. Additionally, the setting of this study was 1 urban catchment area, yielding findings that may not be generalizable to rural settings or urban areas with different population characteristics or policy environments. We also do not know whether police actively targeted areas at greater overdose risk with an incidental frequency that enhanced the appearance of a pattern.

We relied on administrative data that are inherently subject to measurement error. Lack of information about the precise substance and quantity of each seizure or the characteristics of people subject to related enforcement, including association with the drug market as a supplier or consumer, inhibited our ability to explore these factors as potential sources of variation. We do not know whether these results would generalize to an illicit opioid market consisting mainly of analgesics or heroin when estimating dosage under uncertain circumstances. Both substances are much less potent than fentanyl and provide a larger margin of error. We also have no information to inform us of whether there should be a lagged time between seizures based on time to loss of supply, considering that people do not run out of their supply the moment a nearby seizure occurs.

Our measure of nonfatal overdose is also limited because fear of arrest is a well-established deterrent to calling 911 to report an overdose and because community naloxone administration often goes unreported. Certain populations are more likely to administer naloxone themselves or less likely to call 911, especially if previous incidents resulted in incarceration. It is also conceivable that EMS responses vary by neighborhood, that community-level naloxone distribution is affecting results, or that high-profile law enforcement interdiction events may result in a temporarily reduced willingness to call EMS for overdose emergencies. However, these factors would bias our findings toward the null hypothesis, rather than away from it.

Public Health Implications

Our study adds to a growing body of literature that suggests drug criminalization and supply-side interdiction might produce more public harm than public good. This casts doubt on the core assumption of state and federal drug policy and suggests that police officers intending to protect the public's health and safety may be inadvertently exacerbating harms such as fatal overdose. Policymakers need to revisit the role drug policies play in perpetuating an overdose epidemic that is negatively affecting the nation's life expectancy. This should include careful consideration of the population-level consequences from decades of interdiction efforts that have not resulted in any meaningful reduction in the price or availability of drugs in the community over any substantial period and may contribute to increased risk of overdose and its sequelae, including death. AJPH

ABOUT THE AUTHORS

Bradley Ray is with RTI International, Research Triangle Park, NC. Steven J. Korzeniewski is with the School of Medicine, Wayne State University, Detroit, MI. George Mohler is with the Computer Science Department, Boston College, Chestnut Hill, MA. Jennifer J. Carroll is with the Department of Sociology and Anthropology, North Carolina State University, Raleigh. Brandon del Pozo is with the Warren Alpert School of Medicine, Brown University, Providence, RI. Grant Victor is with the School of Social Work, Rutgers University, New Brunswick, NJ. Philip Huynh and Bethany J. Hedden are with the Center for Behavioral Health and Justice, Wayne State University.

CORRESPONDENCE

Correspondence should be sent to Bradley Ray, PhD, RTI International, 3040 Cornwallis Rd, Research Triangle Park, NC 27709 (e-mail: bradleyray@rti.org). Reprints can be ordered at http://www.ajph.org by clicking the "Reprints" link.

PUBLICATION INFORMATION

Full Citation: Ray B, Korzeniewski SJ, Mohler G, et al. Spatiotemporal analysis exploring the effect of law enforcement drug market disruptions on overdose, Indianapolis, Indiana, 2020–2021. *Am J Public Health*. 2023;113(7):750–758.

Acceptance Date: March 13, 2023.

DOI: https://doi.org/10.2105/AJPH.2023.307291

CONTRIBUTORS

B. Ray was the primary investigator. B. Ray and G. Mohler developed the study. S. J. Korzeniewski led the results presentation. J. J. Carroll and B. del Pozo developed hypothesized mechanisms. G. Victor identified extant literature. P. Huynh managed data and provided descriptive statistics. B. J. Hedden managed study protocols and facilitated revisions and idea development for the article. All authors contributed to reviewing and writing drafts and revisions of the article.

ACKNOWLEDGMENTS

This study was funded by the Centers for Disease Control and Prevention (grant 1R01CE003362-01).

We would like to thank Dan O'Donnell and Tom Arkins for identifying the hypothesized mechanism for this study, Meredith Canada for assisting with data acquisition, and Jes Cochran for project consultation. Additionally, we thank the Indianapolis Emergency Medical Services, Marion County Coroner's Office, and the Indianapolis Metropolitan Police Department for providing administrative data sources.

Note. The content of this article is solely the responsibility of the authors and does not necessarily represent the official views of the funders.

CONFLICTS OF INTEREST

The authors have no conflicts of interest to report.

HUMAN PARTICIPANT PROTECTION

This study, including waiver of the Health Insurance Portability and Accountability Act authorization and analysis of limited data sets, was approved by the Wayne State University institutional review board (#21-09-3996).

REFERENCES

1. Ahmad FB, Cisewski JA, Rossen LM, Sutton P. Provisional drug overdose death counts. 2023. Available at: https://www.cdc.gov/nchs/nvss/vsrr/drug-overdose-data.htm. Accessed February 21, 2023.
2. Ciccarone D. The rise of illicit fentanyls, stimulants and the fourth wave of the opioid overdose crisis. *Curr Opin Psychiatry*. 2021;34(4):344–350. https://doi.org/10.1097/YCO.0000000000000717
3. Park JN, Rashidi E, Foti K, Zoorob M, Sherman S, Alexander GC. Fentanyl and fentanyl analogs in the illicit stimulant supply: results from US drug seizure data, 2011–2016. *Drug Alcohol Depend*. 2020;218:108416. https://doi.org/10.1016/j.drugalcdep.2020.108416
4. Holmes LM, Rishworth A, King BH. Disparities in opioid overdose survival and naloxone administration in Pennsylvania. *Drug Alcohol Depend*. 2022;238:109555. https://doi.org/10.1016/j.drugalcdep.2022.109555
5. Lindstrom HA, Clemency BM, Snyder R, Consiglio JD, May PR, Moscati RM. Prehospital naloxone administration as a public health surveillance tool: a retrospective validation study. *Prehosp Disaster Med*. 2015;30(4):385–389. https://doi.org/10.1017/S1049023X15004793
6. Ising A, Proescholdbell S, Harmon KJ, Sachdeva N, Marshall SW, Waller AE. Use of syndromic surveillance data to monitor poisonings and drug overdoses in state and local public health agencies. *Inj Prev*. 2016;22(suppl 1):i43–i49. https://doi.org/10.1136/injuryprev-2015-041821
7. Schell RC, Allen B, Goedel WC, et al. Identifying predictors of opioid overdose death at a neighborhood level with machine learning. *Am J Epidemiol*. 2022;191(3):526–533. https://doi.org/10.1093/aje/kwab279
8. Marks C, Abramovitz D, Donnelly CA, et al. Identifying counties at risk of high overdose mortality burden during the emerging fentanyl epidemic in the USA: a predictive statistical modelling study. *Lancet Public Health*. 2021;6(10):e720–e728. https://doi.org/10.1016/S2468-2667(21)00080-3
9. Bozorgi P, Porter DE, Eberth JM, Eidson JP, Karami A. The leading neighborhood-level predictors of drug overdose: a mixed machine learning and spatial approach. *Drug Alcohol Depend*. 2021;229(pt B):109143. https://doi.org/10.1016/j.drugalcdep.2021.109143
10. Mital S, Wolff J, Carroll JJ. The relationship between incarceration history and overdose in North America: a scoping review of the evidence. *Drug Alcohol Depend*. 2020;213:108088. https://doi.org/10.1016/j.drugalcdep.2020.108088
11. Joudrey PJ, Khan MR, Wang EA, et al. A conceptual model for understanding post-release opioid-related overdose risk. *Addict Sci Clin Pract*. 2019;14(1):17. https://doi.org/10.1186/s13722-019-0145-5
12. Faggiano F, Mathis F, Diecidue R, et al. Opioid overdose risk during and after drug treatment for heroin dependence: an incidence density case–control study nested in the VEdeTTE cohort. *Drug Alcohol Rev*. 2021;40(2):281–286. https://doi.org/10.1111/dar.13173
13. Strang J, McCambridge J, Best D, et al. Loss of tolerance and overdose mortality after inpatient opiate detoxification: follow up study. *BMJ*. 2003;326(7396):959–960. https://doi.org/10.1136/bmj.326.7396.959
14. Mark TL, Parish W. Opioid medication discontinuation and risk of adverse opioid-related health care events. *J Subst Abuse Treat*. 2019;103:58–63. https://doi.org/10.1016/j.jsat.2019.05.001
15. Carroll JJ, Rich JD, Green TC. The protective effect of trusted dealers against opioid overdose in the US. *Int J Drug Policy*. 2020;78:102695. https://doi.org/10.1016/j.drugpo.2020.102695
16. Victor GA, Strickland J, Kheibari A, Flaherty C. A mixed-methods approach to understanding overdose risk-management strategies among a nationwide convenience sample. *Int J Drug Policy*. 2020;86:102973. https://doi.org/10.1016/j.drugpo.2020.102973
17. US Census Bureau. Fastest-growing cities are still in the West and South. May 26, 2022.

Available at: https://www.census.gov/newsroom/press-releases/2022/fastest-growing-cities-population-estimates.html. Accessed June 20, 2022.

18. Rhodes B, Costenbader B, Wilson L, et al. Urban, individuals of color are impacted by fentanyl-contaminated heroin. *Int J Drug Policy.* 2019;73:1–6. https://doi.org/10.1016/j.drugpo.2019.07.008

19. Mohler G, Mishra S, Ray B, et al. A modified two-process Knox test for investigating the relationship between law enforcement opioid seizures and overdoses. *Proc R Soc Math Phys Eng Sci.* 2021;477(2250):20210195. https://doi.org/10.1098/rspa.2021.0195

20. Klauber MR. Two-sample randomization tests for space–time clustering. *Biometrics.* 1971;27(1):129–142. https://doi.org/10.2307/2528932

21. Carter JG, Mohler G, Ray B. Spatial concentration of opioid overdose deaths in Indianapolis: an application of the law of crime concentration at place to a public health epidemic. *J Contemp Crim Justice.* 2019;35(2):161–185. https://doi.org/10.1177/1043986218803527

22. Zibbell JE, Clarke SD, Kral AH, Richardson NJ, Cauchon D, Aldridge A. Association between law enforcement seizures of illicit drugs and drug overdose deaths involving cocaine and methamphetamine, Ohio, 2014–2019. *Drug Alcohol Depend.* 2022;232:109341. https://doi.org/10.1016/j.drugalcdep.2022.109341

23. Zibbell JE, Aldridge AP, Cauchon D, DeFiore-Hyrmer J, Conway KP. Association of law enforcement seizures of heroin, fentanyl, and carfentanil with opioid overdose deaths in Ohio, 2014–2017. *JAMA Netw Open.* 2019;2(11):e1914666. https://doi.org/10.1001/jamanetworkopen.2019.14666

24. Lowder EM, Zhou W, Peppard L, Bates R, Carr T. Supply-side predictors of fatal drug overdose in the Washington/Baltimore HIDTA region: 2016–2020. *Int J Drug Policy.* 2022;110:103902. https://doi.org/10.1016/j.drugpo.2022.103902

25. Rubel SK, Neubert P, Navarretta N, Logan S. Facilitating overdose risk mitigation among patients following a clinician office closure: a Connecticut case study of the opioid rapid response program. *J Public Health Manag Pract.* 2022;28(1, suppl 6):S381–S387. https://doi.org/10.1097/PHH.0000000000001555

26. Acharya JC, Lyons BC, Murthy V, et al. An emergency preparedness response to opioid-prescribing enforcement actions in Maryland, 2018–2019. *Public Health Rep.* 2021;136(1 suppl):9S–17S. https://doi.org/10.1177/00333549211046110

27. del Pozo B, Beletsky L, Goulka J, Kleinig J. Beyond decriminalization: ending the war on drugs requires recasting police discretion through the lens of a public health ethic. *Am J Bioeth.* 2021;21(4):41–44. https://doi.org/10.1080/15265161.2021.1891339

28. Doe-Simkins M, El-Sabawi T, Carroll JJ. Whose concerns? It's time to adjust the lens of research on police-involved overdose response. *Am J Public Health.* 2022;112(9):1239–1241. https://doi.org/10.2105/AJPH.2022.306988

29. Beletsky L, Davis CS. Today's fentanyl crisis: prohibition's iron law, revisited. *Int J Drug Policy.* 2017;46:156–159. https://doi.org/10.1016/j.drugpo.2017.05.050

30. Lambdin BH, Davidson PJ, Browne EN, Suen LW, Wenger LD, Kral AH. Reduced emergency department visits and hospitalisation with use of an unsanctioned safe consumption site for injection drug use in the United States. *J Gen Intern Med.* 2022;37(15):3853–3860. https://doi.org/10.1007/s11606-021-07312-4

31. Betsos A, Valleriani J, Boyd J, Bardwell G, Kerr T, McNeil R. "I couldn't live with killing one of my friends or anybody": a rapid ethnographic study of drug sellers' use of drug checking. *Int J Drug Policy.* 2021;87:102845. https://doi.org/10.1016/j.drugpo.2020.102845

32. Netherland J, Kral AH, Ompad DC, et al. Principles and metrics for evaluating Oregon's innovative drug decriminalization measure. *J Urban Health.* 2022;99(2):328–331. https://doi.org/10.1007/s11524-022-00606-w

33. Pamplin JR II, Rouhani S, Davis CS, King C, Townsend TN. Persistent criminalization and structural racism in US drug policy: the case of overdose good Samaritan laws. *Am J Public Health.* 2023;113(S1):S43–S48. https://doi.org/10.2105/AJPH.2022.307037

34. Network for Public Health Law. 50-State survey. Legal interventions to reduce overdose mortality: overdose good Samaritan laws. Available at: https://www.networkforphl.org/wp-content/uploads/2021/08/2021-50-State-Survey-Legal-Interventions-to-Reduce-Overdose-Mortality-Overdose-Good-Samaritan-Laws-8-18.pdf. Accessed April 9, 2023.

35. Wagner KD, Koch B, Bowles JM, Verdugo SR, Harding RW, Davidson PJ. Factors associated with calling 911 for an overdose: an ethnographic decision tree modeling approach. *Am J Public Health.* 2021;111(7):1281–1283. https://doi.org/10.2105/AJPH.2021.306261

Social Vulnerability in US Communities Affected by Wildfire Smoke, 2011 to 2021

Jason Vargo, PhD, MPH, Brooke Lappe, MPH, Maria C. Mirabelli, PhD, MPH, and Kathryn C. Conlon, PhD, MPH

See also Eisenman, p. 724.

Objectives. To describe demographic and social characteristics of US communities exposed to wildfire smoke.

Methods. Using satellite-collected data on wildfire smoke with the locations of population centers in the coterminous United States, we identified communities potentially exposed to light-, medium-, and heavy-density smoke plumes for each day from 2011 to 2021. We linked days of exposure to smoke in each category of smoke plume density with 2010 US Census data and community characteristics from the Centers for Disease Control and Prevention's Social Vulnerability Index to describe the co-occurrence of smoke exposure and social disadvantage.

Results. During the 2011-to-2021 study period, increases in the number of days of heavy smoke were observed in communities representing 87.3% of the US population, with notably large increases in communities characterized by racial or ethnic minority status, limited English proficiency, lower educational attainment, and crowded housing conditions.

Conclusions. From 2011 to 2021, wildfire smoke exposures in the United States increased. As smoke exposure becomes more frequent and intense, interventions that address communities with social disadvantages might maximize their public health impact. (*Am J Public Health*. 2023;113(7):759–767. https://doi.org/10.2105/AJPH.2023.307286)

AJPH July 2023, Vol 113, No. 7

In recent years, wildfires have, on average, burned more than double the acreage per year compared with earlier decades. In the 1990s, 3.3 million acres were burned per year, while in 2021, 7.1 million acres were burned.[1] Smoke from wildfires compromises air quality by increasing concentrations of particulate matter (PM), ozone, polycyclic aromatic hydrocarbons, volatile organic compounds, and other harmful air pollutants[2–4] that have well-described impacts on respiratory disease and all-cause mortality.[5,6] Projected wildfire trends in the United States predict increasing risk of exposure to wildfire smoke[7] because of increases in weather- and climate-related factors associated with wildfire risk, including heat, drought, and wind speed.[8]

Smoke, also referred to as wildland or wildfire smoke, can travel thousands of miles, potentially exposing distant populations, including communities less prepared for smoke.[9,10] The movement and coverage of wildfire smoke over large areas may result in similar exposures for neighboring communities; however, wildfire risk can vary spatially by population susceptibility and adaptive capacity, or the ability to absorb, recover, and modify exposure to wildfires.[10–15] As with other ambient climate hazards, such as extreme heat, the social and community characteristics that determine adaptive capacity may play an important role in explaining health disparities related to wildfire smoke.[16,17]

Wildfire smoke exposure is associated with asthma exacerbations, chronic obstructive pulmonary disease, respiratory infections, myocardial infarction, ischemic heart disease, heart failure, dysrhythmia, pulmonary embolism, ischemic stroke and transient ischemic attack, out-of-hospital cardiac arrests, and all-cause mortality.[18–20] Public health recommendations to reduce exposure to wildfire smoke currently include recommendations to stay indoors in places with adequate air filtration, reduce activity during smoke events, reduce other sources of indoor air pollution, use air filters, and, for those who cannot stay indoors (e.g., agricultural and outdoor workers),[21] wear suitable respiratory protection when outdoors.[22]

Making these types of changes can be especially difficult for people with limited resources.[11,15,23,24] For example, people without high-quality indoor air filtration at home, those without access to clean air spaces, and people experiencing homelessness might be particularly challenged to make these changes to reduce their personal exposure to wildfire smoke. Recent work shows that wealthier households are more aware of wildfire smoke, allowing them to take protective actions such as closing windows and doors or wearing respirators, seeking out protective devices such as air filters, adjusting their lifestyles to avoid exposures, or more easily temporarily evacuating.[25] Many of the self-protective actions are costly and, therefore, unlikely to benefit some populations.

Demographic, economic, institutional, and sociocultural characteristics such as socioeconomic status, household composition, racial or ethnic minority status, language, and housing type may affect an individual's ability to prepare for, respond to, and recover from wildfire smoke. If these characteristics are associated with an unequal risk of exposure, then these individuals face greater risk of respiratory, cardiovascular, and other adverse health outcomes. We conducted this study to describe wildfire smoke exposure from January 2011 to December 2021 across the United States and to assess the extent to which wildfire smoke exposures overlap with social and community characteristics that might affect adaptive capacity and, as a result, health.

METHODS

We conducted descriptive analyses of the presence of wildfire smoke plumes and their overlap with population centers to describe the magnitude of and trends in wildfire smoke affecting communities across the United States from 2011 to 2021. We combined data on census tract–level wildfire smoke exposures with information about social and community factors, including demographic and socioeconomic components, to characterize wildfire smoke exposures and particularly vulnerable populations.

Wildfire Smoke Exposures

To estimate community-level exposure to wildfire smoke, we combined data from the National Oceanic and Atmospheric Administration Hazard Mapping System (HMS) smoke product[26,27] with population data from the 2010 US Census and American Community Survey.[28] HMS data use satellite-detected fires with multiple daily satellite images and a combination of analyst examination and automated processing to record smoke plumes of categorical densities across North America.[29] Satellite imagery that detects smoke plumes can reliably identify periods of wildland fire influence on ground-level measurements of air quality from validated monitors.[30–32] Plume densities reported in HMS data correlate with $PM_{2.5}$ (particulate matter of ≤ 2.5 microns in diameter) concentrations, with concentrations less than 10 micrograms per cubic meter (μg/m^3) categorized as light, 10 to 21 μg/m^3 as medium, and greater than 21 μg/m^3 as heavy.[27,33]

We assigned daily smoke density categories to each block group center of population and its 2010 population using methods adapted from Vargo.[34] In that work, a block group could be simultaneously assigned plumes of progressively less dense smoke; here, we limited the exposure assignment of each block group on each study day to the densest smoke plume of that day. The resulting quantity, person-days, was the product of the number of people in a census block group and the number of days that block group experiences smoke. We then aggregated person-days by smoke density to the geography and time period of interest for analyses. If any block group in a tract experienced smoke on a given day, we counted that day as a smoke day for the tract. We used census tract person-days in analyses with the other community characteristics.

Social Vulnerability Index

We used the Centers for Disease Control and Prevention's (CDC's) Social Vulnerability Index (SVI) to investigate characteristics that might affect the health risks of wildfire smoke exposures.[35] We conducted all analyses using the 2018 version of the SVI data at the census tract scale. The SVI is a composite index comprising census-derived data on sociodemographic, economic, and cultural characteristics.[35] Flanagan et al.[36] details the methods and data inclusion for the creation of the SVI and SVI components.

Daily person-days of wildfire smoke at the block group level were aggregated to annual census tracts and linked with 2018 SVI percentile rankings of 4 themes: (1) socioeconomic status,

(2) race/ethnicity and language, (3) household composition and disability, and (4) housing and transportation. We estimated person-days and number of smoke-days for each smoke density within tertiles of the distribution of the overall SVI and the 4 component themes. For the housing and transportation theme, which is a household-level index, the resulting quantity was household-days rather than person-days. Hereafter, we refer to the tertiles with the lowest SVI scores as the tertiles with the greatest health and social "advantage" and the tertiles with the highest SVI scores as having the greatest health and social "disadvantage." We assigned tertiles using the census tract file, rather than county-level SVI, to ensure that each of the tertiles represents approximately the same number of people. In addition, we used specific components of the SVI (e.g., the number of persons without a high school diploma) to examine changes in wildfire smoke among specific populations over the study period.

Analytic Methods

We conducted descriptive analyses to describe characteristics of communities in the United States potentially affected by wildfire smoke. For most of these analyses, we compared wildfire smoke estimates in the first 5 years (2011–2015) to those of the last 5 years (2017–2021) of the 11-year study period. Using census tract aggregations of the daily smoke data, we calculated annual numbers of days of each smoke level and used the *t* test to assess changes in the mean frequency of wildfire smoke plumes from the first and last 5 years of the study period; we considered *t* tests with *P* values less than .05 to be statistically significant. In each analysis, we used census tract estimates of person-days as the basis for central tendency estimates within the county or SVI tertile. We performed all analyses with R statistical software.[37]

RESULTS

During the 2011-to-2021 study period, exposure to wildfire smoke increased in the coterminous United States (Figure 1). The total person-days of all categories of wildfire smoke in the last 5 years of the study (2017–2021) increased relative to those in the first 5 years (2011–2015). For heavy-density smoke, the 5-year annual average increased 350%, from 307 million person-days during 2011 to 2015 to 1.381 billion person-days during 2017 to 2021. The increases for light- and medium-density smoke person-days were 39% and 71%, respectively. Counts of person-days by state and smoke density are shown in Tables A1 through A3 (available as supplements to the online version of this article at https://ajph.org).

Most counties in the United States experienced decreases in smoke-free days and increases in days of all smoke densities, with the most pronounced changes for heavy smoke (Figure 2). When we compared the first and last 5 years of the study period, 1517 counties experienced significant decreases in the number of smoke-free days (78.6% of the US population). Similarly, 72.3%, 75.2%, and 87.3% of the population of the United States experienced increases in the number of days of light, medium, and heavy smoke, respectively. The magnitude of the increase in heavy smoke was largest in the western United States (Figure A, available as a supplement to the online version of this article at https://ajph.org). While western states of Idaho, Oregon, and Washington experienced 339%, 340%, and 297% increases in heavy smoke days per year, respectively, the eastern states of Maryland, South Carolina, and Virginia also experienced substantial increases (166%, 88%, and 233%, respectively).

Census tracts in the highest SVI tertile (i.e., tracts at the greatest overall disadvantage for living healthy lives) experienced a 358% increase in the average annual number of heavy smoke days, from 0.92 (95% confidence interval [CI] = 0.91, 0.93) days in 2011 to 2015 to 4.21 (95% CI = 4.18, 4.25) days in 2017 to 2021. We observed similar increases for the SVI's 4 themes: (1) socioeconomic status: 346%; (2) race/ethnicity and language: 449%; (3) household composition and disability: 309%; and (4) housing and transportation: 357%.

Table B (available as a supplement to the online version of this article at https://ajph.org) shows the average annual number of days in each of the SVI themes and tertiles. The coincidence of heavy smoke person-days with highest overall SVI percentile occurred primarily in the American West and north along the Canadian border (Figure B, available as a supplement to the online version of this article at https://ajph.org). Notably, 3 states—California, Oregon, and Washington—accounted for 39% of the heavy smoke person-days in the highest SVI tertile. The average number of days of all smoke densities in tracts at the highest SVI tertile increased significantly between the start and end of the study period. However, tracts with the highest SVI tertile did not account for a disproportionate amount of all heavy smoke person-days. Rather, each tertile of SVI tracts was evenly distributed.

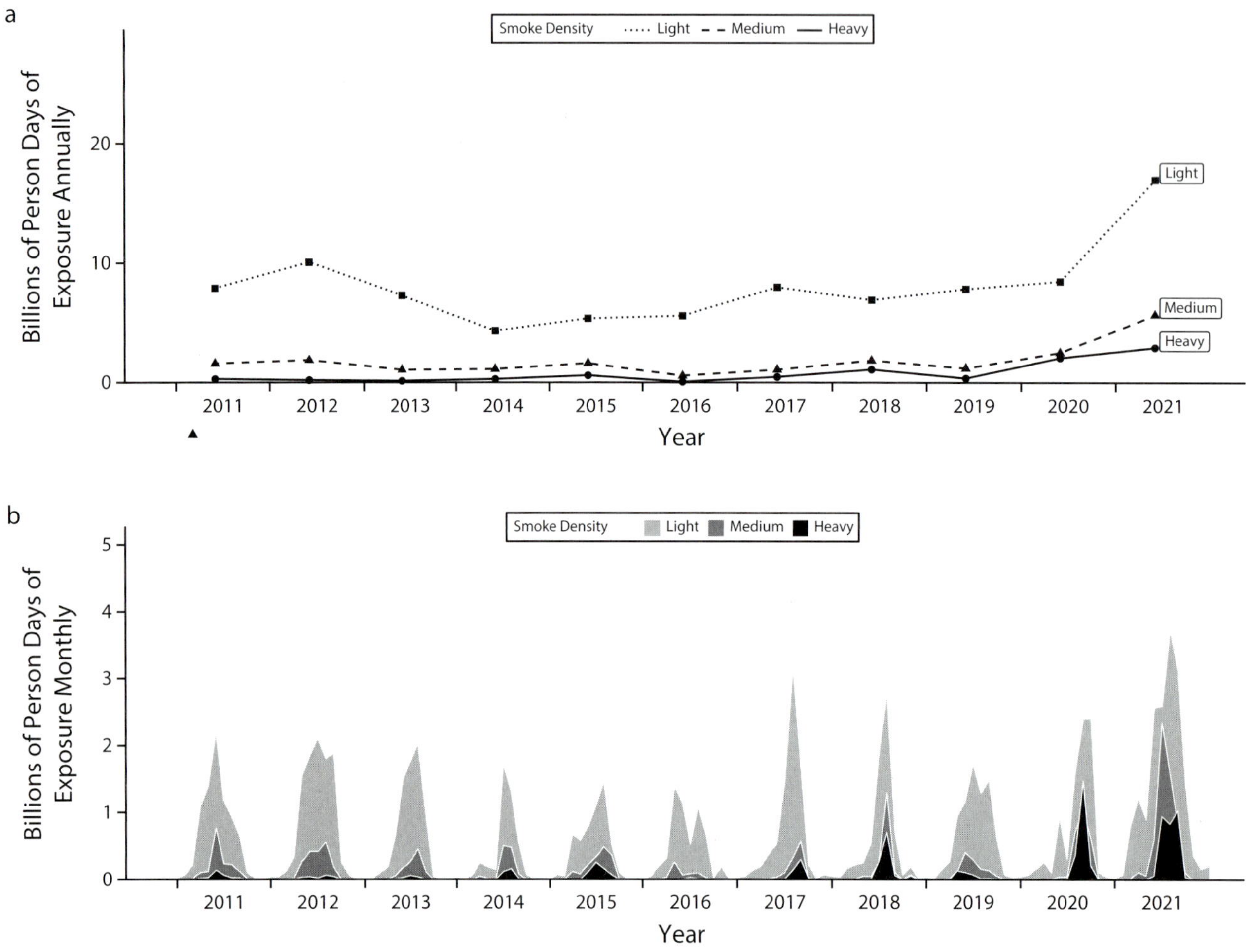

FIGURE 1— Potential Wildfire Smoke Exposure in the United States by Smoke Density and (a) Year and (b) Month: 2011–2021

Person-days of smoke varied across specific SVI components. When we compared the first and last 5 years of the study period, the percentage increases in person- (or household-) days differed by SVI component (Figure 3). Increases were observed among all components, with the largest increases seen for heavy-density plumes. Components of the SVI's race/ethnicity/language theme, including minority populations and individuals with limited English proficiency, exhibited some of the largest increases; for example, the minority component in the race/ethnicity/language theme had the largest increase in number of person-days for any SVI component across all smoke densities (Figure C, available as a supplement to the online version of this article at https://ajph.org). Notable increases were also seen for components such as crowded households and multifamily housing from the housing and transportation theme. Tracts with the highest number of persons in these components and themes tend to be more concentrated in the western United States,[35] relative to the rest of the United States and, thus, overlap with the largest smoke exposure increases in the study (Figure A).

DISCUSSION

Person-days of exposure to light, medium, and heavy wildfire smoke in the United States increased significantly from 2011 to 2021, but the most pronounced change was seen for heavy smoke (Figure 1). Exposures to smoke were not distributed equally, and the increases in smoke were largest in the most disadvantaged communities. This is especially concerning given that wildfire smoke exposure is associated with a number of negative respiratory and cardiovascular health effects.[18–20] Health outcomes such as cardiovascular disease and cerebrovascular emergency department visits have been linked specifically to heavy-density smoke exposure.[20] Our findings suggest that individuals living in communities with limited resources to reduce

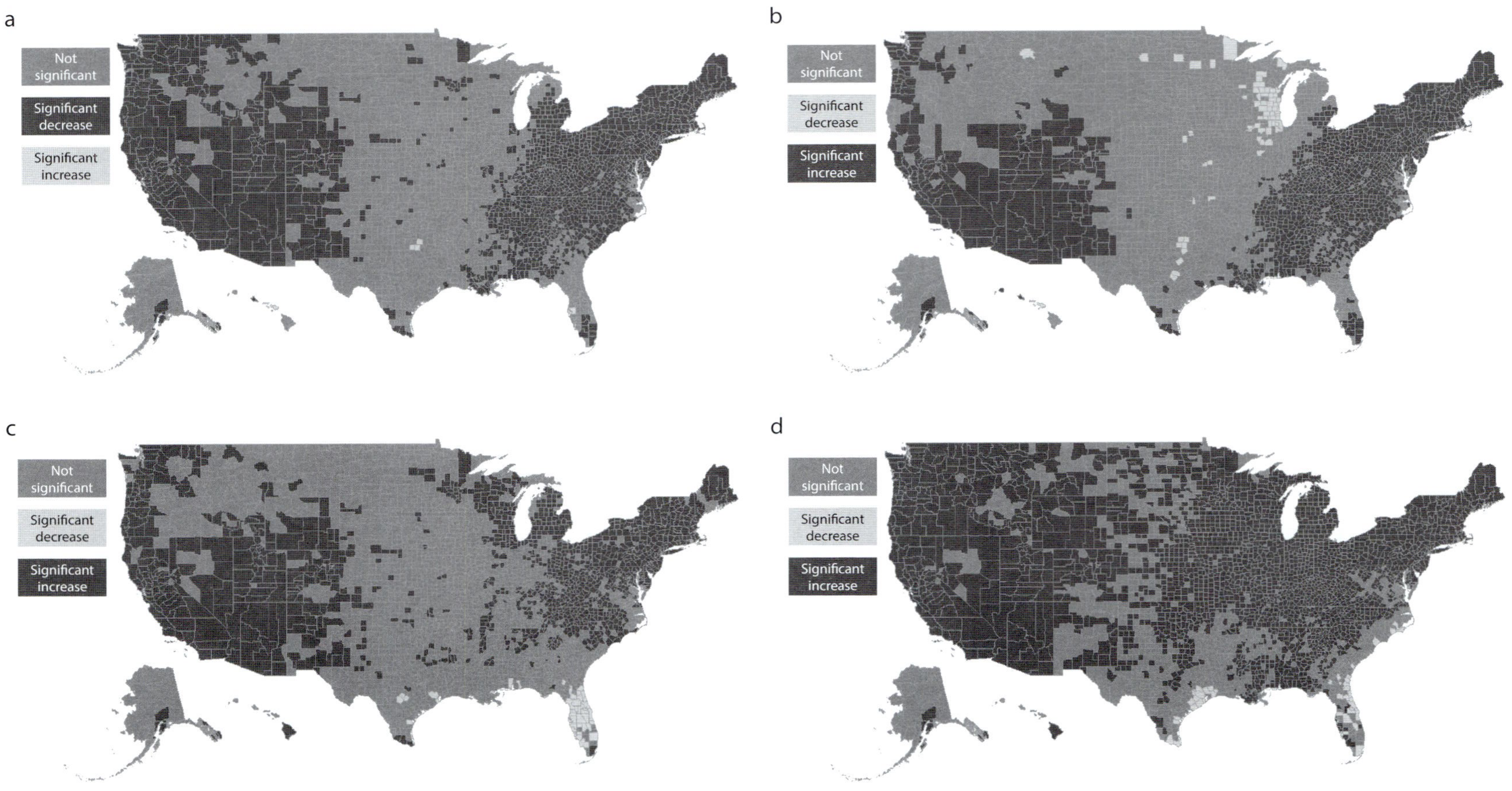

FIGURE 2— Counties With Significant Changes in the Number of Days (a) Without Wildfire Smoke, (b) With Light Wildfire Smoke, (c) With Medium Wildfire Smoke, and (d) With Heavy Wildfire Smoke: United States, 2011–2015 vs 2017–2021

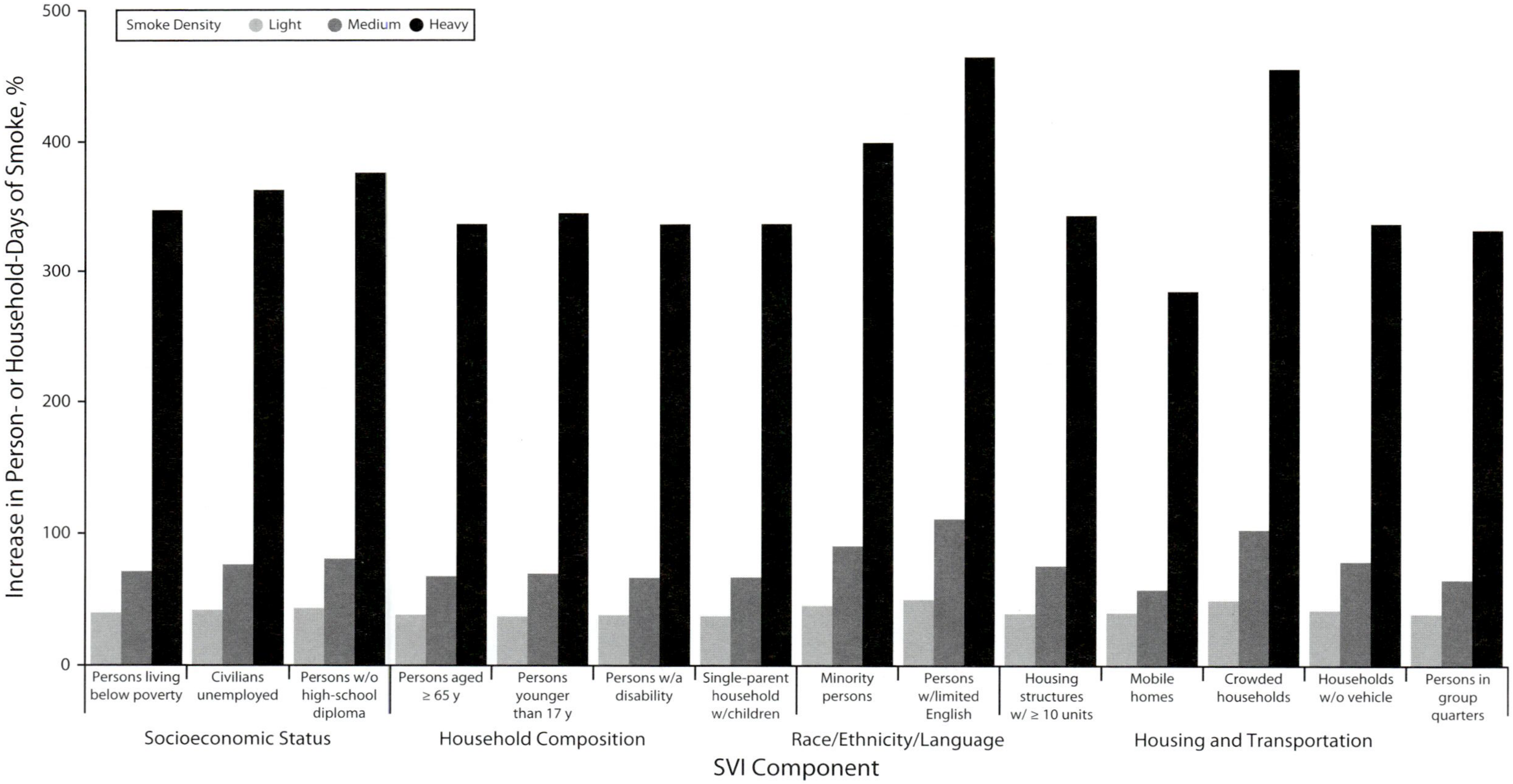

FIGURE 3— Percentage Change in Person- or Household-Days of Wildfire Smoke Exposure by Social Vulnerability Index (SVI) Theme: United States, 2011–2015 to 2017–2021

the health impacts of the smoke exposures have seen the frequency of such exposures increase dramatically across this study's time period.

We estimated an annual average increase of approximately 1 billion person-days of heavy smoke and medium smoke, and more than 2.5 billion person-days for light smoke. These estimates might represent an upper bound for potential wildfire smoke–exposed populations, in part because populations move between census tracts over time. Also, HMS data are derived from satellite plume data rather than ground-level measurements of air quality. A recent analysis of the air quality monitor record covering a much longer study period estimated that wildfires and meteorology led to increased harmful air pollution exposures by 25 million person-days annually over the last 20 years.[7] Nonetheless, the trends observed here are important for public health planning because even more conservative estimates of wildfire smoke exposures than those presented here would produce significant health impacts and costs to individuals and health care systems. A national study estimated that Americans are willing to pay $129 per day to avoid the health impacts of being exposed to heavy smoke, indicating the social and economic costs of wildfires.[38]

Broadly speaking, the characteristics of people or a community (e.g., age, race, health status, income), social inequalities (e.g., social capital, political power, lack of access to information), place-based inequalities (e.g., rural vs urban, elevation), and adaptation inequalities[39] combine to affect a population's susceptibility to disaster events and their resulting impacts. Our findings suggest that increases in smoke are occurring in communities with the highest disadvantage. Individual components of the SVI may be associated with both increased susceptibility to wildfire and decreased adaptive capacity.[40] The SVI does not include every indicator that may be desired to capture susceptibility to wildfire smoke; however, as a composite of several social determinants of health, it may serve as a sufficient proxy in the absence of better, more specific data.

If the adaptive capacity is hindered by factors such as the language in which wildfire warning systems deliver messages, then those with the highest disadvantage in the race/ethnicity and language theme may be the most impacted. Similarly, opportunities to reduce exposures are affected by existing housing not being fitted with proper air filtration or other smoke prevention measures, which may be more common in older multiunit houses, mobile homes, or crowded housing considered under the highest housing and transportation disadvantage. Communities with fewer economic resources as indicated by highest SVI may face more barriers in avoiding outdoor exposures following a wildfire smoke event.[40]

While we assessed social disadvantage and wildfire smoke, vulnerability as captured by the SVI is relevant to a wider range of climate-related disasters including more proximate exposure to wildfire and its effects.[10,41–43] Social vulnerability and adaptive capacity affect the ability to prepare for and recover from the fire, evacuation, or clean up. Wildfires present difficult recovery trajectories for communities with housing and transportation disadvantage because of the enormous destruction of housing supply, which makes it more difficult to find adequate housing, especially in the high-cost regions of the West.[44,45]

More than 71.8 million properties face some risk of wildfires over the next 30 years, representing an immense challenge to future housing security.[46] Communities with low SVI have more resources to build and rebuild at high wildfire-risk areas such as the wildland urban interface,[11] whereas communities with high SVI often have less. Repeated shocks and stresses of wildfires can push individuals living in communities with high SVI into a permanent state of poverty[47] and perpetuate a cycle of disparities. However, this overlap of social vulnerability and growing exposure suggests that interventions that consider housing modifications, such as retrofits and air purification, particularly in communities with high SVI, may more effectively reduce the potential health impacts and social and economic losses associated with wildfire smoke.

While we did find that the highest SVI tertile in the housing and transportation theme had one of the highest increases in smoke exposure days, this theme falls short of including the people especially susceptible to smoke exposure: people experiencing homelessness. People experiencing homelessness face a lack of regular shelter, access to information, and resources to prepare and respond to wildfires, which amplify their wildfire smoke and health risk.[48–50] A 2020 survey of people experiencing homelessness in Portland, Oregon, found that 75% did not receive any information during wildfires, and 69% received no type of help during wildfire and smoke events.[51] Spare and less-reliable data on persons experiencing homelessness prevent a detailed accounting of smoke exposures among such persons; however, the states in which wildfire smoke exposure is the highest are the same states in which the population of persons experiencing homelessness is growing the fastest.[52] As areas at the wildland–urban interface

AJPH July 2023, Vol 113, No. 7

continue to be occupied by people with differing susceptibility, intensifying wildfires are likely to prompt discussions on who will be most affected by wildfires and how to address related injustices and social equity concerns.

In this study, we used the CDC's SVI to provide information about the demographic, economic, institutional, and sociocultural characteristics of census tracts in the coterminous United States. The SVI is based on publicly available data and does not explicitly account for numerous factors affecting exposure to wildfire smoke or the burden of its associated health effects, but has been correlated with increased prevalence of several pre-existing conditions that exacerbate adverse health outcomes associated with smoke exposures.[53,54] Because the SVI values are representative of a community, rather than any one individual in that community, it may misclassify individuals who are represented by an SVI ranking that is not indicative of their personal social advantages.

HMS data cannot differentiate plumes of differing heights in the atmosphere; thus, a plume may be over a census tract with minimal impact on ground-level air quality. Studies examining the correlation between plume presence and monitored air quality have shown significant increases in $PM_{2.5}$, particularly in the presence of medium and heavy smoke plume.[32] The HMS data do not differentiate sources of fire smoke; smoke from prescribed fires are included in smoke estimations. However, fires of the size and intensity typical of prescribed burns are less likely to result in heavy smoke plumes. Our analysis focuses mostly on heavy smoke because it is expected to be the most detrimental for health and is increasing most for most of the population.

Our data show that wildfire smoke exposure coincides with demographic, economic, institutional, and sociocultural characteristics. Our results suggest that there are inequalities in wildfire smoke exposures by SVI and highlight opportunities to identify geographic areas in need of increased emergency preparedness messages, supplies, shelters, and recovery support. These findings can be used by emergency planners and others to better understand and address the contribution of wildfire smoke to poor health. Designing and implementing specific interventions for communities experiencing economic and social disadvantage may improve health in communities and for individuals exposed to wildfire smoke in a changing climate. AJPH

ABOUT THE AUTHORS

Jason Vargo is with the Federal Reserve Bank of San Francisco, San Francisco, CA. Brooke Lappe is a doctoral student in the Gangarosa Department of Environmental Health, Rollins School of Public Health, Emory University, Atlanta, GA. Maria C. Mirabelli is with the Asthma and Community Health Branch, Division of Environmental Health Science and Practice, National Center for Environmental Health, Centers for Disease Control and Prevention, Atlanta, GA. Kathryn C. Conlon is with the Department of Public Health Sciences, School of Medicine, and the Department of Veterinary Medicine and Epidemiology, School of Veterinary Medicine, University of California Davis.

CORRESPONDENCE

Correspondence should be sent to Jason Vargo, PhD, Federal Reserve Bank of San Francisco, 101 Market St., San Francisco, CA 94105 (e-mail: jason.vargo@sf.frb.org). Reprints can be ordered at https://ajph.org by clicking the "Reprints" link.

PUBLICATION INFORMATION

Full Citation: Vargo J, Lappe B, Mirabelli MC, Conlon KC. Social vulnerability in US communities affected by wildfire smoke, 2011 to 2021. *Am J Public Health*. 2023;113(7):759–767.

Acceptance Date: March 10, 2023.

https://doi.org/10.2105/AJPH.2023.307286

CONTRIBUTORS

J. Vargo contributed to conceptualizing the study, conducted data management and processing of wildfire smoke information and the Social Vulnerability Index, and contributed to the methods, analysis, interpretation of results, and writing of the article. B. Lappe led the writing and revising of the article and contributed to interpretation of results. M. C. Mirabelli conceptualized the study and contributed to interpretation of results and writing and revision of the article. K. C. Conlon contributed to conceptualizing the study, method selection, interpretation of results, and revision of the article. All authors approved submission of the article to be published.

CONFLICTS OF INTEREST

All authors have no conflicts of interest to declare.

HUMAN PARTICIPANT PROTECTION

No protocol approval was needed for this study because the data used were publicly available, deidentified, and obtained from secondary sources.

REFERENCES

1. Hoover K, Hanson LA. Wildfire statistics. CRS In Focus, IF10244. Washington, DC: Library of Congress, Congressional Research Service; 2022.
2. Andreae MO, Merlet P. Emission of trace gases and aerosols from biomass burning. *Global Biogeochem Cycles*. 2001;15(4):955–966. https://doi.org/10.1029/2000GB001382
3. Carabali G, Villanueva-Macias J, Ladino LA, et al. Characterization of aerosol particles during a high pollution episode over Mexico City. *Sci Rep*. 2021;11(1):22533. https://doi.org/10.1038/s41598-021-01873-4
4. Langmann B, Duncan B, Textor C, Trentmann J, van der Werf GR. Vegetation fire emissions and their impact on air pollution and climate. *Atmos Environ*. 2009;43(1):107–116. https://doi.org/10.1016/j.atmosenv.2008.09.047
5. Cascio WE. Wildland fire smoke and human health. *Sci Total Environ*. 2018;624:586–595. https://doi.org/10.1016/j.scitotenv.2017.12.086
6. Rappold AG, Reyes J, Pouliot G, Cascio WE, Diaz-Sanchez D. Community vulnerability to health impacts of wildland fire smoke exposure. *Environ Sci Technol*. 2017;51(12):6674–6682. https://doi.org/10.1021/acs.est.6b06200
7. Kalashnikov DA, Schnell JL, Abatzoglou JT, Swain DL, Singh D. Increasing co-occurrence of fine particulate matter and ground-level ozone extremes in the western United States. *Sci Adv*. 2022;8(1):eabi9386. https://doi.org/10.1126/sciadv.abi9386
8. Xu R, Yu P, Abramson MJ, et al. Wildfires, global climate change, and human health. *N Engl J Med*. 2020;383(22):2173–2181. https://doi.org/10.1056/NEJMsr2028985
9. Afrin S, Garcia-Menendez F. Potential impacts of prescribed fire smoke on public health and socially vulnerable populations in a Southeastern US state. *Sci Total Environ*. 2021;794:148712. https://doi.org/10.1016/j.scitotenv.2021.148712

10. Palaiologou P, Ager AA, Nielsen-Pincus M, Evers CR, Day MA. Social vulnerability to large wildfires in the western USA. *Landsc Urban Plan.* 2019; 189:99–116. https://doi.org/10.1016/j.landurbplan.2019.04.006
11. Davies IP, Haugo RD, Robertson JC, Levin PS. The unequal vulnerability of communities of color to wildfire. *PLoS One.* 2018;13(11):e0205825. https://doi.org/10.1371/journal.pone.0205825
12. Gaither CJ, Goodrick S, Murphy BE, Poudyal N. An exploratory spatial analysis of social vulnerability and smoke plume dispersion in the US South. *Forests.* 2015;6(5):1397–1421. https://doi.org/10.3390/f6051397
13. Paveglio TB, Brenkert-Smith H, Hall T, Smith AMS. Understanding social impact from wildfires: advancing means for assessment. *Int J Wildland Fire.* 2015;24(2):212–224. https://doi.org/10.1071/WF14091
14. Paveglio TB, Edgeley CM, Stasiewicz AM. Assessing influences on social vulnerability to wildfire using surveys, spatial data and wildfire simulations. *J Environ Manage.* 2018;213:425–439. https://doi.org/10.1016/j.jenvman.2018.02.068
15. Wigtil G, Hammer RB, Kline JD, et al. Places where wildfire potential and social vulnerability coincide in the coterminous United States. *Int J Wildland Fire.* 2016;25(8):896–908. https://doi.org/10.1071/WF15109
16. Eisenman DP, Wilhalme H, Tseng C-H, et al. Heat death associations with the built environment, social vulnerability and their interactions with rising temperature. *Health Place.* 2016;41: 89–99. https://doi.org/10.1016/j.healthplace.2016.08.007
17. Basu R, Ostro BD. A multicounty analysis identifying the populations vulnerable to mortality associated with high ambient temperature in California. *Am J Epidemiol.* 2008;168(6):632–637. https://doi.org/10.1093/aje/kwn170
18. Reid CE, Brauer M, Johnston FH, Jerrett M, Balmes JR, Elliott CT. Critical review of health impacts of wildfire smoke exposure. *Environ Health Perspect.* 2016;124(9):1334–1343. https://doi.org/10.1289/ehp.1409277
19. Heaney A, Stowell JD, Liu JC, Basu R, Marlier M, Kinney P. Impacts of fine particulate matter from wildfire smoke on respiratory and cardiovascular health in California. *GeoHealth.* 2022;6(6): e2021GH000578. https://doi.org/10.1029/2021GH000578
20. Wettstein ZS, Hoshiko S, Fahimi J, Harrison RJ, Cascio WE, Rappold AG. Cardiovascular and cerebrovascular emergency department visits associated with wildfire smoke exposure in California in 2015. *J Am Heart Assoc.* 2018;7(8):e007492. https://doi.org/10.1161/JAHA.117.007492
21. Navarro K. Working in smoke: wildfire impacts on the health of firefighters and outdoor workers and mitigation strategies. *Clin Chest Med.* 2020; 41(4):763–769. https://doi.org/10.1016/j.ccm.2020.08.017
22. Stone S, Anderko L, Berger M, et al. *Wildfire Smoke: A Guide for Public Health Officials, Revised 2019.* EPA/452/R-19/901. Washington, DC: US Environmental Protection Agency, Office of Research and Development; 2019.
23. Collins TW. What influences hazard mitigation? Household decision making about wildfire risks in Arizona's White Mountains. *Prof Geogr.* 2008; 60(4):508–526. https://doi.org/10.1080/00330120802211737
24. Collins TW, Bolin B. Situating hazard vulnerability: people's negotiations with wildfire environments in the US southwest. *Environ Manage.* 2009;44(3): 441–455. https://doi.org/10.1007/s00267-009-9333-5
25. Burke M, Heft-Neal S, Li J, et al. Exposures and behavioural responses to wildfire smoke. *Nat Hum Behav.* 2022;6(10):1351–1361. https://doi.org/10.1038/s41562-022-01396-6
26. Justice CO, Giglio L, Korontzi S, et al. The MODIS fire products. *Remote Sens Environ.* 2002;83(1–2): 244–262. https://doi.org/10.1016/S0034-4257(02)00076-7
27. Hazard Mapping System Fire and Smoke Product—product information. National Oceanic and Atmospheric Administration, Office of Satellite and Product Operations. Available at: https://www.ospo.noaa.gov/Products/land/hms.html#about. Accessed May 11, 2023.
28. Design and methodology: American Community Survey. Washington, DC: US Census Bureau; 2010.
29. Ruminski M, Simko J, Kibler J, et al. Use of multiple satellite sensors in NOAA's operational near real-time fire and smoke detection and characterization program. Vol 7089. Bellingham, WA: SPIE; 2008.
30. Larsen AE, Reich BJ, Ruminski M, Rappold AG. Impacts of fire smoke plumes on regional air quality, 2006–2013. *J Expo Sci Environ Epidemiol.* 2018;28(4):319–327. https://doi.org/10.1038/s41370-017-0013-x
31. Shrestha PM, Humphrey JL, Carlton EJ, et al. Impact of outdoor air pollution on indoor air quality in low-income homes during wildfire seasons. *Int J Environ Res Public Health.* 2019;16(19):3535. https://doi.org/10.3390/ijerph16193535
32. Preisler HK, Schweizer D, Cisneros R, Procter T, Ruminski M, Tarnay L. A statistical model for determining impact of wildland fires on particulate matter ($PM_{2.5}$) in central California aided by satellite imagery of smoke. *Environ Pollut.* 2015;205: 340–349. https://doi.org/10.1016/j.envpol.2015.06.018
33. Knapp KR, Frouin R, Kondragunta S, Prados A. Toward aerosol optical depth retrievals over land from GOES visible radiances: determining surface reflectance. *Int J Remote Sens.* 2005; 26(18):4097–4116. https://doi.org/10.1080/01431160500099329
34. Vargo JA. Time series of potential US wildland fire smoke exposures. *Front Public Health.* 2020;8: 126. https://doi.org/10.3389/fpubh.2020.00126
35. Centers for Disease Control and Prevention/Agency for Toxic Substances and Disease Registry/Geospatial Research, Analysis, and Services Program. CDC/ATSDR Social Vulnerability Index 2018, US database. Available at: https://www.atsdr.cdc.gov/placeandhealth/svi/data_documentation_download.html. Accessed December 2021.
36. Flanagan BE, Gregory EW, Hallisey EJ, Heitgerd JL, Lewis B. A social vulnerability index for disaster management. *J Homel Secur Emerg Manag.* 2011; 8(1):3. https://doi.org/10.2202/1547-7355.1792
37. R Core Team. R: A language and environment for statistical computing. Vienna, Austria: R Foundation for Statistical Computing; 2021.
38. Jones BA. Willingness to pay estimates for wildfire smoke health impacts in the US using the life satisfaction approach. *J Environ Econ Policy.* 2018;7(4):403–419. https://doi.org/10.1080/21606544.2018.1463872
39. Cutter S, Boruff B, Shirley W. Social vulnerability to environmental hazards. *Soc Sci Q.* 2003;84(2): 242–261. https://doi.org/10.1111/1540-6237.8402002
40. Murphy DJ, Wyborn C, Yung L, Williams DR. Key concepts and methods in social vulnerability and adaptive capacity. Gen Tech Rep RMRS-GTR-328. Fort Collins, CO: US Department of Agriculture, Forest Service, Rocky Mountain Research Station; 2015:328.
41. Morrow BH. Identifying and mapping community vulnerability. *Disasters.* 1999;23(1):1–18. https://doi.org/10.1111/1467-7717.00102
42. Juntunen L. *Addressing Social Vulnerability to Hazards.* Eugene, OR: University of Oregon Eugene; 2004.
43. Rodríguez H, Quarantelli EL, Dynes RR, Andersson WA, Kennedy PA, Ressler E. *Handbook of Disaster Research.* Vol 643. New York, NY: Springer; 2007. https://doi.org/10.1007/978-0-387-32353-4
44. Comerio MC. *Disaster Hits Home: New Policy for Urban Housing Recovery.* Oakland, CA: University of California Press; 1998. https://doi.org/10.1525/9780520918726
45. Settembrino MR. Hurricane Sandy's impact on the predisaster homeless and homeless shelter services in New Jersey. *J Emerg Manag.* 2016; 14(1):7–16. https://doi.org/10.5055/jem.2016.0268
46. Porter J. The construction of probabilistic wildfire risk estimate for individual real estate parcels for the contiguous United States. *Fire.* 2022;5(4):117. https://doi.org/10.3390/fire5040117
47. Ibarraran ME, Ruth M. Climate change and natural disasters: Economic and distributional impacts. In: *Distributional Impacts of Climate Change and Disasters.* Cheltenham, UK: Edward Elgar Publishing; 2009. https://doi.org/10.4337/9781849802338.00010
48. Every D, Thompson K. Disaster resilience: can the homeless afford it? *Aust J Emerg Manag.* 2014;29(3):52–56.
49. Gin JL, Balut MD, Der-Martirosian C, Dobalian A. Managing the unexpected: the role of homeless service providers during the 2017–2018 California wildfires. *J Community Psychol.* 2021;49(7):2532–2547. https://doi.org/10.1002/jcop.22653
50. Gin JL, Levine CA, Canavan D, Dobalian A. Including homeless populations in disaster preparedness, planning, and response: a toolkit for practitioners. *J Public Health Manag Pract.* 2022;28(1):E62–E72. https://doi.org/10.1097/PHH.0000000000001230
51. Hines M, Petteni M, Knowlton S, Roots S. Stories from the Outside: Oregon Wildfires 2020. Portland State Homelessness Research & Action Collaborative. 2021. Available at: https://pdxscholar.library.pdx.edu/cgi/viewcontent.cgi?article=1029&context=hrac_pub. Accessed May 4, 2023.
52. US Department of Housing and Urban Development. The 2020 annual homeless assessment report (AHAR) to Congress (Part 1: Point-in-time-estimates of homelessness). January 2021. Available at: https://www.huduser.gov/portal/sites/default/files/pdf/2020-AHAR-Part-1.pdf. Accessed May 4, 2023.
53. Park E, Ko Y. Socioeconomic Vulnerability Index and obesity among Korean adults. *Int J Environ Res Public Health.* 2021;18(24):13370. https://doi.org/10.3390/ijerph182413370
54. Flanagan BE, Hallisey EJ, Adams E, Lavery A. Measuring community vulnerability to natural and anthropogenic hazards: the Centers for Disease Control and Prevention's Social Vulnerability Index. *J Environ Health.* 2018;80(10):34–36.

Stratified Simple Random Sampling Versus Volunteer Community-Wide Sampling for Estimates of COVID-19 Prevalence

Rachel J. Keith, PhD, Rochelle H. Holm, PhD, Alok R. Amraotkar, MD, Megan M. Bezold, J. Michael Brick, PhD, Adrienne M. Bushau-Sprinkle, PhD, Krystal T. Hamorsky, PhD, Kathleen T. Kitterman, MS, Kenneth E. Palmer, PhD, Ted Smith, PhD, Ray Yeager, PhD, and Aruni Bhatnagar, PhD

See also Elliott, p. 721.

AJPH July 2023, Vol 113, No. 7

Objectives. To evaluate community-wide prevalence of severe acute respiratory syndrome coronavirus 2 (SARS-CoV-2) infection using stratified simple random sampling.

Methods. We obtained data for the prevalence of SARS-CoV-2 in Jefferson County, Kentucky, from adult random (n = 7296) and volunteer (n = 7919) sampling over 8 waves from June 2020 through August 2021. We compared results with administratively reported rates of COVID-19.

Results. Randomized and volunteer samples produced equivalent prevalence estimates ($P < .001$), which exceeded the administratively reported rates of prevalence. Differences between them decreased as time passed, likely because of seroprevalence temporal detection limitations.

Conclusions. Structured targeted sampling for seropositivity against SARS-CoV-2, randomized or voluntary, provided better estimates of prevalence than administrative estimates based on incident disease. A low response rate to stratified simple random sampling may produce quantified disease prevalence estimates similar to a volunteer sample.

Public Health Implications. Randomized targeted and invited sampling approaches provided better estimates of disease prevalence than administratively reported data. Cost and time permitting, targeted sampling is a superior modality for estimating community-wide prevalence of infectious disease, especially among Black individuals and those living in disadvantaged neighborhoods. (*Am J Public Health*. 2023;113(7):768–777. https://doi.org/10.2105/AJPH.2023.307303)

Accurate estimates of disease prevalence are a prerequisite for evaluating the spread of infectious diseases and for mounting appropriately scaled and targeted public health responses. Since John Snow's tracking to prove his hypothesis, appropriate approaches to the surveillance of community rates of infection have been a matter of ongoing public health debate.[1] More recently, many approaches have been proposed, the most rigorous of which involve probability and nonprobability sampling.[2–7] In the United States, estimates of the prevalence of local and imported infectious diseases are based on the National Notifiable Diseases Surveillance System, while many chronic conditions are estimated from a self-reported phone survey.[8,9] There have been few, if any, attempts to estimate ongoing disease prevalence using stratified simple random sampling, and the utility and biases of this approach remain unclear, vis-à-vis other modes of sampling.

During the recent COVID-19 pandemic, large-scale spread of infections necessitated rapid and timely estimates of prevalence. However, only administratively reported data were available. Early in the pandemic, testing was limited, but even when it became widely available, it relied on nonprobability sampling, which was disproportionately inaccessible to marginalized communities[10] and likely to be biased because of a higher probability of voluntary testing by individuals suspecting infections or, in contrast, not seeking testing to avoid quarantine. Most health surveys had to modify their collection programs because of the pandemic.[11] Although randomized sampling was used to estimate the prevalence of infection in California, Georgia, Indiana, Oregon, and Rhode Island,[12–15] these surveys have limitations in sample size or spatial and temporal resolution and did not provide estimates of the reliability and the biases inherent to this approach. Hence, for improved public health response, we developed evidence-based estimates of community-wide prevalence based on stratified simple randomized sampling and compared this with convenience sampling and administratively reported cases.

METHODS

Our study took place in 8 waves between June 2020 and August 2021.

Probability Sampling

To estimate the prevalence of SARS-CoV-2 infections in Jefferson County, Kentucky, we conducted stratified simple random sampling (Table 1). Participants were residents aged 18 years or older. Study procedures included self-report electronic surveys to collect information on demographics, occupation, contact and risk, health history, lifestyle, COVID-19 vaccination (as applicable), and wastewater monitoring awareness (for wave 8 only) as well as professional collection of nasal swabs and blood samples.

For recruitment, we divided the county into 4 geographic zones (Figure 1) guided by census tract lines to reflect distinctly different demographics (age, race, income, education, and population density). We integrated local knowledge to keep intact macro-neighborhoods encompassing similar cultural identity often delineated along physical geographic boundaries. Zones included at least 100 000 residents.

For the recruitment of the probability sample, we selected households using the address-based sampling frame derived from US Postal Service delivery files.[16] For each wave, we mailed 18 000 to 36 000 invitations across the county (Appendix A, Figure A1, available as a supplement to the online version of this article at http://ajph.org). We divided the county into 8 sampling strata, where each of the 4 zones was split in half. We allocated the sample approximately equally to each strata to provide reliable estimates by stratum.

We determined the total number sampled for each wave based on the time and funds required to send out invitations between waves and response rates from previous waves. For the samples from the first 4 waves, we deduplicated them so each address could only be sampled once during these 4 waves. For the fifth wave, we selected an independent sample, and for the subsequent waves, we deduplicated the samples so each household could only be sampled once in waves 5 through 8. It is possible a household

TABLE 1— Demographic Characteristics and Percentage of Antibody-Positive Participants in the Probability and Volunteer Samples for Waves 1 Through 8: Jefferson County, KY, June 2020–August 2021

	Probability (Waves 1–8)		Volunteer (Waves 1–8)	
Characteristic	No. (Weighted %)	Positive Antibody (Weighted %)	No. (Weighted %)	Positive Antibody (Weighted %)
Total	7296 (100.0)	13.2	7919 (100.0)	14.1
Female	4363 (59.8)	12.9	4981 (62.9)	12.6
White	6271 (86.0)	12.7	6489 (81.9)	12.2
Age, y				
18–34	891 (12.2)	14.2	1463 (18.5)	11.6
35–59	2706 (37.1)	12.4	3655 (46.2)	12.6
≥ 60	3699 (50.7)	13.4	2801 (35.4)	13.5
Single family home	6293 (86.3)	13.4	6813 (86.0)	12.3
Smoker	574 (7.9)	8.5	595 (7.5)	8.3
E-cigarette user	181 (2.5)	14.1	219 (2.8)	12.5
Chronic conditions	3924 (53.8)	13.9	3607 (45.5)	13.2
COVID-19 symptoms	438 (6.0)	17.5	725 (9.2)	12.4

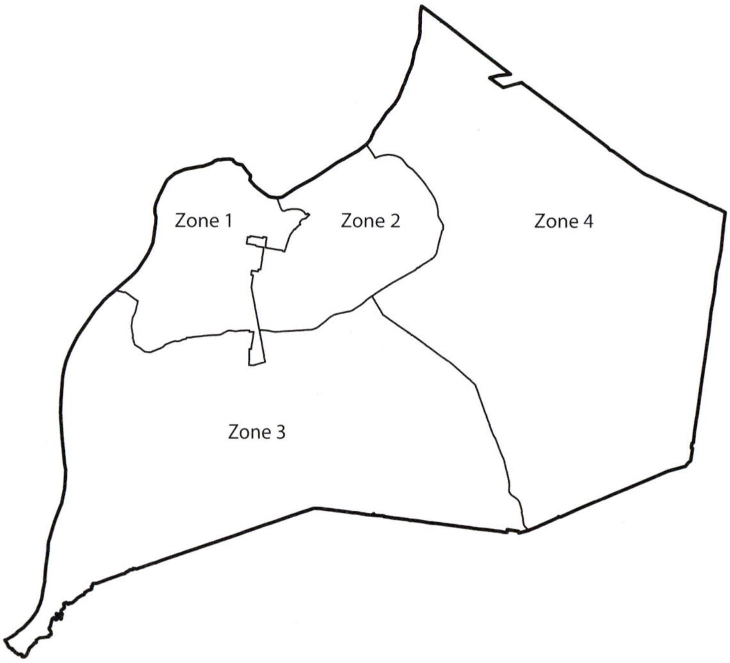

		Age, Years, %				Sex, %		Race, %	
Zone	Adults, No.	18–24	25–44	45–64	≥ 65	Male	Female	White	People of Color
Total	594 943	11.2	35.1	34.0	19.8	47.5	52.5	74.8	25.2
1	97 055	15.8	34.3	36.0	13.8	46.2	53.8	39.2	60.8
2	100 029	13.7	39.5	29.4	17.4	47.9	52.1	89.5	10.5
3	206 589	12.2	37.5	33.4	16.8	47.9	52.1	76.3	23.7
4	191 270	8.7	34.7	36.3	20.3	47.6	52.4	83.8	16.2

FIGURE 1— Sampling Zones and Demographic Characteristics Within Jefferson County, KY

AJPH July 2023, Vol 113, No. 7

could have been sampled once in waves 1 to 4 and sampled again once in waves 5 to 8. When we sampled a household, one adult was randomly selected to participate. For waves 7 and 8, we redefined the strata by wastewater treatment plant sewershed, but we aggregated the results back to the original strata. An invitation to participate in the study was mailed to the address, and we asked the sampled adult to go to a Web site to complete an English screening interview and schedule a testing appointment. Community partners provided incentives in waves 5 and 6.

Our weighting steps included adjustments for (1) sampling the household from the stratum, (2) sampling 1 adult within the household, and (3) adjusting the estimated totals (raking) to the number of adults in the county from the American Community Survey[17] tabulations (the 2018 5-year data file). The first 2 weighting steps accounted for the probability of selection. The primary goal of the raking was to adjust for nonresponse. The 3 raking dimensions were sex by age, race, and zone. There were no other data on the sampling frame that could reduce nonresponse bias. If any weights were too large, they were trimmed, and the weights were raked again to match the control totals. For variance estimation, we created 50 jackknife replicate weights for each wave.[18] We used these replicate weights to estimate the standard errors and 95% confidence intervals. The raking may reduce the nonresponse in the estimates but cannot eliminate it.

Volunteer Sampling

For the volunteer sample, social media, community outreach, press conferences, and news outlets, as well as personal contacts with influential community members, were used to invite community participants to sign up online and come to a testing facility. Those who walked up without previously signing up online were also accommodated.

Individuals who consented for testing but were not part of the probability sample were designated "volunteers." To produce estimates from this sample, we assigned respondents an initial weight of 1 and then raked using the same procedures used for the probability sample. We also created replicate weights to estimate precision, assuming the volunteer sample was equivalent to a simple random sample within the 4 zones. The raking may reduce nonresponse bias but relies on model assumptions that rarely hold in practice.

Testing

Convenient testing dates and times were available for participants to come to drive-up collection sites spread throughout the 4 zones over about 5 days during each wave of testing. Probability and volunteer participants both had trained staff collect nasopharyngeal swabs, which were analyzed for current infection by reverse transcription polymerase chain reaction (RT-PCR) and blood finger-prick samples for the presence of SARS-CoV-2–specific antibodies by serological assessment (enzyme-linked immunoabsorbent assay [ELISA]). Previous exposure to SARS-CoV-2 was assessed via ELISA by measuring immunoglobulin G (IgG) responses to SARS-CoV-2 antigens spike (S), spike receptor binding domain, and nucleocapsid (N) proteins.[19] The presence of IgG to N is highly indicative of natural infection, whereas the presence of IgG to S could be attributable to natural infection or vaccination. The SARS-CoV-2 vaccines were made widely available to the public in Kentucky starting in April 2021. For waves 1 through 4 (June 2020 through February 2021) and for unvaccinated participants in waves 5 through 8 (April through August 2021), previous exposure to SARS-CoV-2 was determined by presence versus absence of S IgG antibodies in peripheral blood samples. From April through August 2021, for vaccinated participants, previous exposure was determined via presence of N IgG and absence of any self-reported disease or COVID-19–related symptoms before sampling.

Prevalence

To produce prevalence estimates, we made adjustments for sensitivity and specificity depending on the participant's vaccination status. If the participant reported they were not vaccinated, then we made the same adjustments as for the initial period based on the highly reliable S-protein ELISA. The sensitivity of the S-protein ELISA is 100.0 and the specificity is 98.8. If the participant was vaccinated, then we adjusted the estimates for the sensitivity (65.0) and specificity (85.0) of the N-protein test. The test for the N-protein was not available in wave 4; thus, we excluded the 120 vaccinated participants in that wave from our analysis.

Because of the very different measurement properties of the tests, the adjustments should be noted.[20] For example, if the observed prevalence rate was 10.0%, then the adjusted estimate would be 10.18% if it were based on the S-protein but 20.0% if based on the N-protein. All estimates of prevalence reported were adjusted unless stated otherwise (Appendix B, available as a supplement to the online version of this article at http://ajph.org).

Administratively Reported Data

Administrative data from July 2020 to August 2021 from the Jefferson County health authority, Louisville Metro Public Health and Wellness, are publicly available. Administrative data for June 2020 are set to zero. We conducted geocoding to the study zones using ArcGIS Pro version 2.8.0 (Esri, Redlands, CA; Appendix C, available as a supplement to the online version of this article at http://ajph.org).

Decay

Respondents infected early in 2020 might not still show a positive antibody response if tested in mid-2021 because of seropositivity decay. One approach to make the estimates more comparable is to adjust the administrative statistics to account for the decay in seropositivity at the point of time of the testing and whether the participant was vaccinated or not.[21] In essence, this approach transforms the administrative estimates of prevalence into estimates of seropositivity, and we refer to the regression estimate of positivity as the "decayed" administrative estimate.

Statistical Analysis

Study data were collected and managed using Research Electronic Data Capture (REDCap) tools hosted at the University of Louisville[22,23] before being transferred to SAS version 9.4 (SAS Institute Inc, Cary, NC) for data curation and analysis.[18] We computed the estimates and their standard errors using the final and replicate weights using PROC SurveyFreq to account for the complex sample design. The weighting was important in producing the prevalence estimates (before any measurement error adjustments) as the median absolute difference in the estimates for the probability sample was 1.8 percentage points. The analysis used either the t test or χ^2 test of significance.

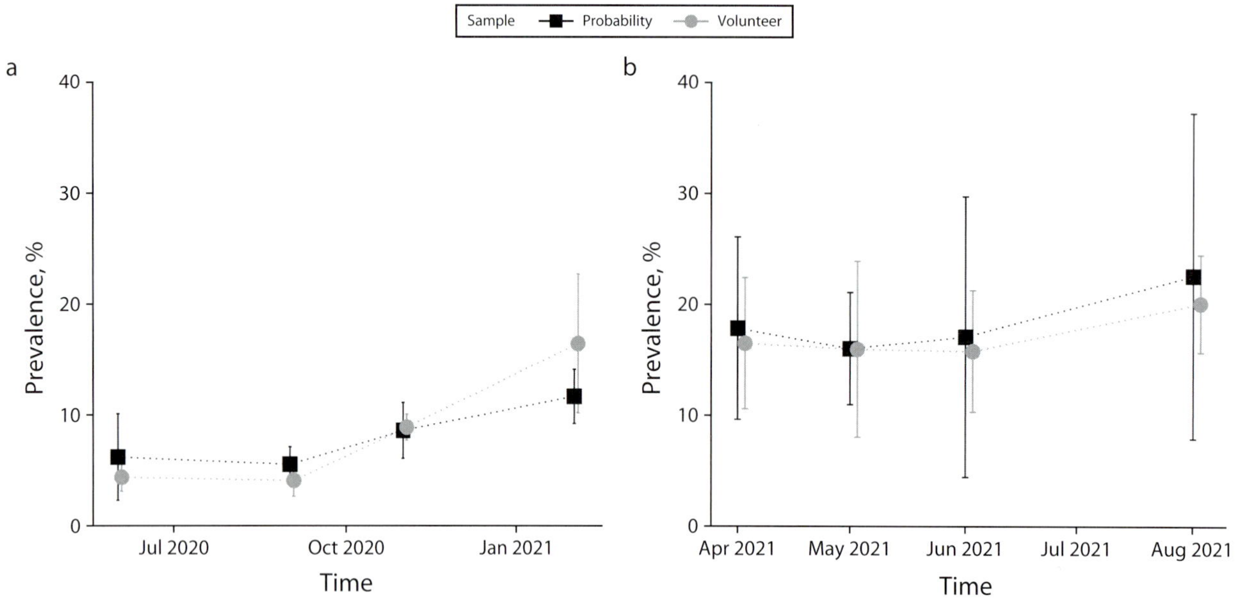

FIGURE 2— Prevalence Estimates for Probability and Volunteer Participants Who Tested Positive for SARS-CoV-2 Infections for (a) Waves 1–4 and (b) Waves 5–8: Jefferson County, KY, June 2020–August 2021

Note. IgG = immunoglobulin G; SARS-CoV-2 = severe acute respiratory syndrome coronavirus 2. Vertical lines represent 95% confidence intervals. Waves 1–4 in panel a present participants positive for SARS-CoV-2 spike (S) protein–specific IgG antibodies. Waves 5–8 in panel b present unvaccinated participants positive for SARS-CoV-2 S protein–specific IgG antibodies and vaccinated participants positive for SARS-CoV-2 nucleocapsid (N)–specific IgG antibodies and absence of any self-reported previous infection or related symptoms before sampling.

RESULTS

Over the 8 waves, most individuals in the probability sample were White (86%) and aged older than 35 years (88%), while 60% were female; the volunteer sample had a similar demographic distribution (Table 1). Distribution was highly clustered to the urban core of the county (Appendix A, Figure A2, available as a supplement to the online version of this article at http://ajph.org). Weighting attempted to compensate for these differences. Although we collected nasopharyngeal samples to detect active infections, the low positivity rates observed precluded their use in the analysis. Prevalence estimates in the following sections are, thus, based on positive antibodies. The adult participants in the probability and volunteer samples reported being vaccinated against COVID-19 at a high rate, 90% by August 2021, which is substantially higher than the nearly 62% total county-wide residents who had received a first vaccine dose by that time.

The response rate for the probability sample (percentage of the sampled cases tested) ranged from 2.4% to 5.5% over the 8 waves. Recruitment of a representative study sample posed a significant challenge throughout the project. The exception was wave 8 (August 2021) with higher prevailing public concern about infection levels during the B.1.617.2 (Delta) surge compared with the original (wild-type) SARS-CoV-2 and its subsequent variants. We also scheduled wave 8 by using prediction modeling from community wastewater sampling,[24] which allowed approximation of the Delta variant surge dates. The response rate was higher for both invited and volunteer study participants during wave 8.

Probability and Volunteer Prevalence

The estimated prevalence estimates from the probability and volunteer samples were comparable ($P > .05$) for each of the first 4 waves (Figure 2a; Appendix A, Figure A3, available as a supplement to the online version of this article at http://ajph.org). We examined prevalence estimates by other characteristics including age, sex, race, smoker status, e-cigarette use, chronic conditions, symptoms, and county zone, and the probability and volunteer estimates did not differ substantially ($P > .05$). For waves 5 through 8, the probability and volunteer prevalence estimates were also similar ($P > .05$;

Figure 2b); estimates by other characteristics again did not differ substantially during this period ($P > .05$), with only 1 of 10 differences being statistically significant. Because these 2 sources produced similar estimates, we combined them to produce composite estimates that were based on larger sample sizes and had greater precision. We created the composites separately for each of the 8 waves by weighting the estimates for each source by the number of observations and dividing by the total number of observations. We computed the variances by weighting in the proportion of the observations in the source.

Composite and Administrative Prevalence

The composite estimates of prevalence for waves 1 through 4 showed little variation for men (7.0%) versus women (7.1%), for those with (6.9%) or without (7.2%) chronic conditions, and for e-cigarette users (7.0%) versus nonusers (7.0%). However, White (6.3%) versus Black (9.2%) persons with a difference of −3.0% (−4.8% to −1.2%) and smokers (2.4%) versus nonsmokers (7.4%) with a difference of −5.1% (−7.2% to −2.9%) showed diversity.

Early in the pandemic, the estimated prevalence estimates based on compositing the estimate were higher than from administrative sources ($P < .001$ for waves 1 through 4). The composite estimate was, on average, 11 percentage points higher than administrative sources across these 4 waves (Appendix A, Figure A4, available as a supplement to the online version of this article at http://ajph.org), but there were some differences in the populations covered. One difference is the administrative sources included all persons regardless of age. Restricting the administrative source estimate to adults would shift the estimate up only approximately 0.5 percentage points and does not alter the conclusion that the administrative sources underestimated the prevalence rate. When we compared the composite estimates of prevalence for waves 1 through 4 with county administrative sources, the difference for men versus women was small (–0.2 compared with 0.5) but the difference for White versus Black (–3.0 compared with −0.1) was substantial. The administrative data indicated a lower rate of infection for Black individuals than our composite estimate.

For waves 5 through 8, the administrative estimates were closer to the composite estimates, and some of the differences were no longer statistically significant. The administrative statistics exhibited the expected monotone increasing pattern for prevalence, while the composite estimates dipped after February before rising again in August 2021. Because prevalence should be monotonically increasing over time, this dip may be attributable to a decay in the seropositivity of those infected earlier.[21]

When further analyzed for the 4 geographic zones (Figure 3), composite estimates were often higher than the administrative estimates. The sample precision to estimate population differences at this level of disaggregation was low, and the differences were not statistically significant at the .05 level.

Temporal Estimates

The decayed administrative estimate differed only slightly from the unadjusted administrative estimate until wave 5 (April 2021) when the difference was more substantial (Appendix A, Figure A4, available as a supplement to the online version of this article at http://ajph.org). When we compared the decayed administrative estimate to the composite estimate for April through June 2021, we observed the earlier pattern with the composite estimate being higher for every wave, except wave 7, when the difference was not statistically significant (for the other waves all the differences had $P < .05$). The decayed administrative estimate was sharply lower than the composite for August 2021 when the peak percentage of participants' SARS-CoV-2 prevalence was 21%, almost 5 percentage points higher than the June 2021 estimate. The administrative data had a lower increase in reported cases during this period (1.9%) and was less than increases in both February 2021 (4.5%) and November 2020 (2.2%).

DISCUSSION

These unique data from a large study, unduplicated elsewhere, beginning within months of the pandemic emergence, enabled us to faithfully follow the pandemic trajectory and to assess the relative efficacy of different sampling approaches for estimating the community-wide prevalence of infection. We also recognized that probability sampling only would not provide accurate modeling opportunities and that not allowing volunteer participation when COVID-19 testing was limited would have been unethical in an emergency public health crisis. Still, the response rate varied from wave to wave. The limitations with low-prevalence diseases were also corroborated when probability-based sampling of active infections was used for households for HIV.[25]

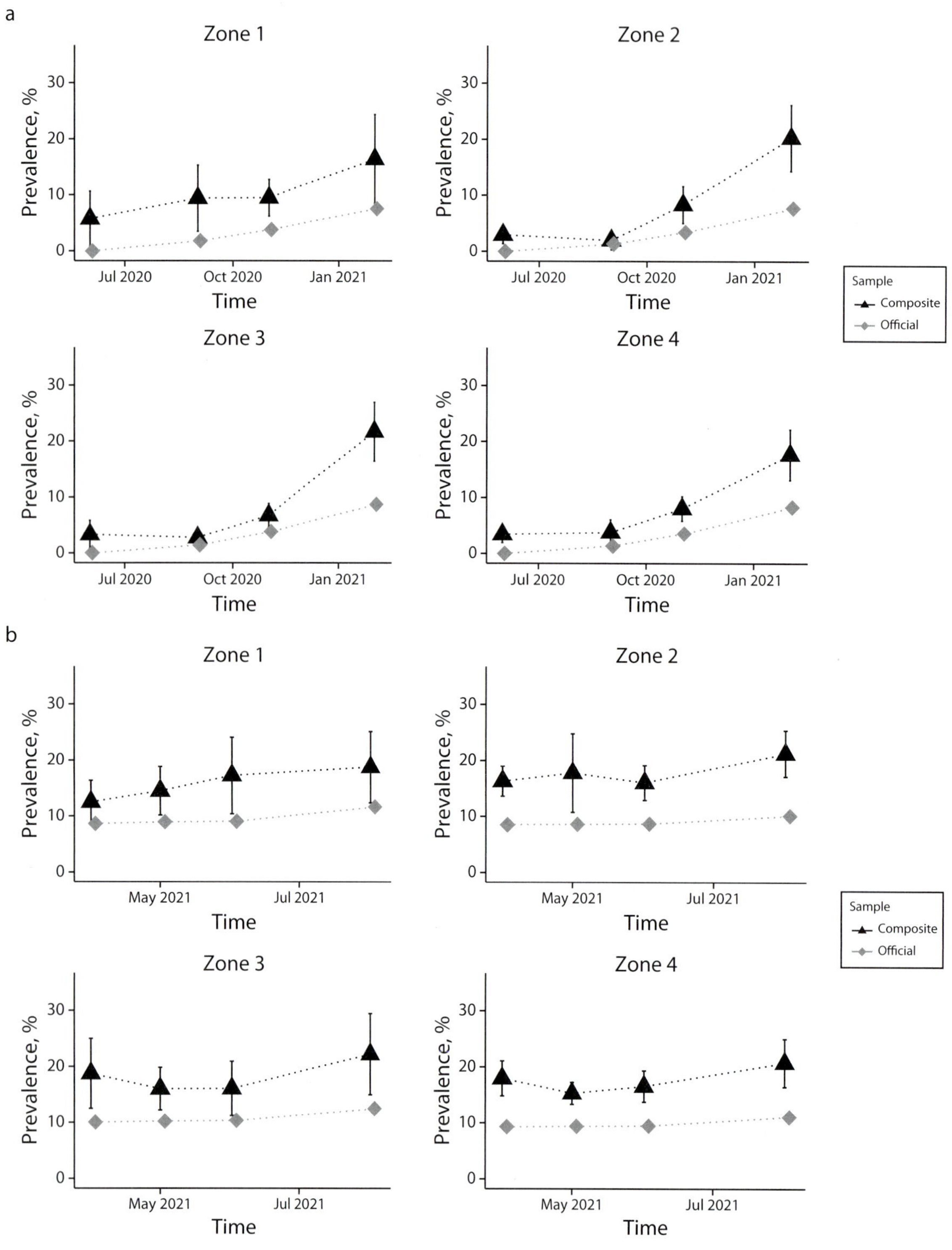

FIGURE 3— Prevalence Estimates for a Composite of Probability and Volunteer Participants Who Tested Positive for SARS-CoV-2 Infections and Administratively Reported Official Rates by Geographic Zones for (a) Waves 1–4 and (b) Waves 5–8: Jefferson County, KY, June 2020–August 2021

Note. IgG = immunoglobulin G; SARS-CoV-2 = severe acute respiratory syndrome coronavirus 2. Administratively reported data are from the Jefferson County health authority, Louisville Metro Public Health and Wellness. Vertical lines represent 95% confidence intervals. Waves 1–4 in panel a present participants positive for SARS-CoV-2 spike (S) protein–specific IgG antibodies and administratively reported official rates. Waves 5–8 in panel b present unvaccinated participants positive for SARS-CoV-2 spike (S) protein–specific IgG antibodies and vaccinated participants positive for SARS-CoV-2 nucleocapsid (N)–specific IgG antibodies and absence of any self-reported previous infection or related symptoms before sampling and administratively reported official rates.

We did not find substantive differences between the prevalence estimates from the volunteer and probability samples by wave. This might be somewhat surprising because self-selection bias in volunteer samples in social and behavioral sciences research has long been considered a serious problem,[5] although the contribution of these biases may vary.[2,7] We found even within serological convenience versus random sampling studies there was no clear concurrence, with no substantive differences in vaccine-preventable diseases in schoolchildren,[3] while nontyphoid *Salmonella* infections had large differences.[4] Unique to our study, during the pandemic, large amounts of unverified information being shared through social networks[26] might have contributed to selection bias. For example, an invited or volunteer participant would need to be interested in testing to seek out participation, and those who did not believe in COVID-19 or its adverse consequences would not sample regardless of invitation type.

Our low response rate for the probability samples (less than 6%) may result in a nonresponse bias similar to the self-selection bias in the volunteer sample estimates. Virtually all face-to-face surveys collecting physical specimens suspended operations during this time,[27] and at the beginning of this pandemic, there were few to no treatment options. So, our study is important in the context of how to recruit participants in a pandemic to support community-related public health and not optimize individual health. Probability sample response rates less than 30% are susceptible to substantial bias.[28] Our experience suggests that the probability sample is not likely to produce estimates with lower bias unless methods for increasing the response rate can be implemented.

Although our volunteer and probability samples gave similar estimates of prevalence, it does not follow they were both unbiased. In both, the percentage who were vaccinated was much higher than county-level estimates. Moreover, even though our sample sizes were too small to detect differences in the 4 county zones, we did see variance in the administrative data per wave, which would suggest that other cities that utilized convenience sampling[10] may also have underreported spatial inequities. Finally, the similarity between the probability and nonprobability sampling results may be because of the high prevalence of the disease and the large number of individuals tested (several thousand), which may have led to similar estimates of disease prevalence, regardless of the sampling approach.

In our analysis, we also aimed to understand the relationship between the tested samples and the administrative statistics as a comparator for sampling methods. Our composite sample has some precedent; it is similar to use of other probability and volunteer hybrid prevalence estimators for HIV[29] and in substance use and mental health outcomes.[6] In our initial period before vaccinations, the composite estimates were consistently between 2- and 4-fold higher than estimates from administrative records. These results suggest that, on a national level, the rates of SARS-CoV-2 infections may have been at least 2-fold higher than previously estimated. We also found statistical differences of the composite estimates of prevalence for waves 1 through 4 for White and minority respondents, and both our probability and volunteer samples had a significantly higher number of minority participants than in administrative records. This is consistent with the disproportionate impact of the pandemic on minorities.[30] Our study suggests that effective outreach improves participation of underserved or marginalized populations.

Waves 5 through 8 were more complicated, relying largely on data from the less reliable N-protein test. This meant that administrative seroprevalence (decayed) estimates were lower than the composite prevalence estimates. However, these adjustments reduce data comparability. If our conclusion that both the probability and volunteer samples are underestimates of prevalence holds, then the administrative statistics underestimate the prevalence to a greater extent than our comparisons show.

Limitations

While the major strength of our study was the longitudinal testing, results are limited by low participation. The low response rates for the probability sample could have introduced biases that could not be eliminated by the weighting. Moreover, because of the availability of vaccines, the antibody testing procedures had to be modified, and the sensitivity and specificity of the tests were vastly different. To help address these issues, we first analyzed the data from June 2020 to February 2021, before most vaccinations and substantial decrease in seropositivity over time, then we analyzed at the later period (through August 2021) as an attempt to compensate for the vaccination and time differences. We assumed that a positive antibody test result could be from 1 or more times of infection. Lastly, while volunteers may have been altruistic for public health research, they may have enrolled because they thought they had COVID-19.

Public Health Implications

In our study, we found that administrative reports of positive cases during the COVID-19 pandemic underestimated the actual prevalence, which in the early stages of the pandemic may have been 2- to 4-fold higher than reported. Although stratified simple random sampling was superior to administrative record keeping, its efficacy was similar to convenient, invited sampling. Both approaches were limited by a low response rate. Nonetheless, targeted sampling by invitation led to greater participation of the Black population. These findings underscore the importance of community outreach in improving participation in testing and other public health interventions. AJPH

ABOUT THE AUTHORS

Rachel J. Keith, Rochelle H. Holm, Alok R. Amraotkar, Ted Smith, Ray Yeager, and Aruni Bhatnagar are with the Christina Lee Brown Envirome Institute, School of Medicine, University of Louisville, Louisville, KY. Megan M. Bezold, Adrienne M. Bushau-Sprinkle, Krystal T. Hamorsky, Kathleen T. Kitterman, and Kenneth E. Palmer are with the Center for Predictive Medicine for Biodefense and Emerging Infectious Diseases, University of Louisville. J. Michael Brick is with Westat Inc, Rockville, MD.

CORRESPONDENCE

Correspondence should be sent to Aruni Bhatnagar, Christina Lee Brown Envirome Institute, School of Medicine, University of Louisville, 302 E Muhammad Ali Blvd, Louisville, KY 40202 (e-mail: aruni.bhatnagar@louisville.edu). Reprints can be ordered at http://ajph.org by clicking the "Reprints" link.

PUBLICATION INFORMATION

Full Citation: Keith RJ, Holm RH, Amraotkar AR, et al. Stratified simple random sampling versus volunteer community-wide sampling for estimates of COVID-19 prevalence. *Am J Public Health*. 2023; 113(7):768–777.

Acceptance Date: March 20, 2023.

DOI: https://doi.org/10.2105/AJPH.2023.307303

CONTRIBUTORS

R. J. Keith and R. H. Holm are joint first authors. All authors participated in the design and study investigation. J. M. Brick conducted data analyses, and all authors reviewed analysis results. R. H. Holm drafted the article. All authors edited and approved the final article.

ACKNOWLEDGMENTS

This work was supported by contracts from the Centers for Disease Control and Prevention (GB210585) and the Louisville–Jefferson County Metro Government as a component of the Coronavirus Aid, Relief, and Economic Security Act, as well as grants from the James Graham Brown Foundation, the Owsley Brown II Family Foundation, and the Welch Family. Reverse transcription polymerase chain reaction diagnostics for waves 1 to 4 and serology work were also supported in part by the Jewish Heritage Fund and the Center for Predictive Medicine for Biodefense and Emerging Infectious Disease.

Note. The funding sources had no role in the study design; data collection; administration of the interventions; analysis, interpretation, or reporting of data; or decision to submit the findings for publication.

CONFLICTS OF INTEREST

The authors report no relevant competing interests.

HUMAN PARTICIPANT PROTECTION

For the seroprevalence and data on severe acute respiratory syndrome coronavirus 2–infected individuals provided by Louisville Metro Public Health and Wellness under a data transfer agreement, the University of Louisville institutional review board (IRB) approved this as human participant research (IRB: 20.0393). Both participant groups consented to agree to participate in the research and provided electronic or written informed consent.

REFERENCES

1. Snow J. *Mode of Communication of Cholera*. 2nd ed. London, England: John Churchill; 1855.
2. Hultsch DF, MacDonald SW, Hunter MA, Maitland SB, Dixon RA. Sampling and generalisability in developmental research: comparison of random and convenience samples of older adults. *Int J Behav Dev*. 2002;26(4):345–359. https://doi.org/10.1080/01650250143000247
3. Kelly H, Riddell MA, Gidding HF, Nolan T, Gilbert GL. A random cluster survey and a convenience sample give comparable estimates of immunity to vaccine preventable diseases in children of school age in Victoria, Australia. *Vaccine*. 2002; 20(25–26):3130–3136. https://doi.org/10.1016/S0264-410X(02)00255-4
4. Emborg HD, Simonsen J, Jørgensen CS, et al. Seroincidence of non-typhoid *Salmonella* infections: convenience vs. random community-based sampling. *Epidemiol Infect*. 2016;144(2):257–264. https://doi.org/10.1017/S0950268815001417
5. Cheung KL, Peter M, Smit C, de Vries H, Pieterse ME. The impact of non-response bias due to sampling in public health studies: a comparison of voluntary versus mandatory recruitment in a Dutch national survey on adolescent health. *BMC Public Health*. 2017;17(1):276. https://doi.org/10.1186/s12889-017-4189-8
6. Drabble LA, Trocki KF, Korcha RA, Klinger JL, Veldhuis CB, Hughes TL. Comparing substance use and mental health outcomes among sexual minority and heterosexual women in probability and non-probability samples. *Drug Alcohol Depend*. 2018;185:285–292. https://doi.org/10.1016/j.drugalcdep.2017.12.036
7. Krueger EA, Fish JN, Hammack PL, Lightfoot M, Bishop MD, Russell ST. Comparing national probability and community-based samples of sexual minority adults: implications and recommendations for sampling and measurement. *Arch Sex Behav*. 2020;49(5):1463–1475. https://doi.org/10.1007/s10508-020-01724-9
8. Centers for Disease Control and Prevention. National Notifiable Diseases Surveillance System (NNDSS). Available at: https://www.cdc.gov/nndss/index.html. Accessed May 25, 2022.
9. Pickens CM, Pierannunzi C, Garvin W, Town M. Surveillance for certain health behaviors and conditions among states and selected local areas—Behavioral Risk Factor Surveillance System, United States, 2015. *MMWR Surveill Summ*. 2018;67(9): 1–90. https://doi.org/10.15585/mmwr.ss6709a1
10. Bilal U, Tabb LP, Barber S, et al. Spatial inequities in COVID-19 testing, positivity, confirmed cases, and mortality in 3 US cities: an ecological study. *Ann Intern Med*. 2021;174(7):936–944. https://doi.org/10.7326/M20-3936
11. Ward BW, Sengupta M, DeFrances CJ, Lau DT. COVID-19 pandemic impact on the national health care surveys. *Am J Public Health*. 2021; 111(12):2141–2148. https://doi.org/10.2105/AJPH.2021.306514
12. Menachemi N, Yiannoutsos CT, Dixon BE, et al. Population point prevalence of SARS-CoV-2 infection based on a statewide random sample—Indiana, April 25–29, 2020. *MMWR Morbid Mortal Wkly Rep*. 2020;69(29):960–964. https://doi.org/10.15585/mmwr.mm6929e1
13. Chan PA, King E, Xu Y, et al. Seroprevalence of SARS-CoV-2 antibodies in Rhode Island from a statewide random sample. *Am J Public Health*. 2021;111(4):700–703. https://doi.org/10.2105/AJPH.2020.306115
14. Layton BA, Kaya D, Kelly C, et al. Evaluation of a wastewater-based epidemiological approach to estimate the prevalence of SARS-CoV-2 infections and the detection of viral variants in disparate Oregon communities at city and neighborhood scales. *Environ Health Perspect*. 2022;130(6):67010. https://doi.org/10.1289/EHP10289
15. Sullivan PS, Siegler AJ, Shioda K, et al. Severe acute respiratory syndrome coronavirus 2 cumulative incidence, United States, August 2020–December 2020. *Clin Infect Dis*. 2022;74(7):1141–1150. https://doi.org/10.1093/cid/ciab626
16. Iannacchione VG. The changing role of address-based sampling in survey research. *Public Opin Q*. 2011;75(3):556–575. https://doi.org/10.1093/poq/nfr017
17. US Census Bureau. 2018 American Community Survey (ACS). US Department of Commerce. Available at: https://www.census.gov/data/developers/data-sets/acs-5year.html. Accessed June 21, 2021.

18. Rust KF, Rao JN. Variance estimation for complex surveys using replication techniques. *Stat Methods Med Res.* 1996;5(3):283–310. https://doi.org/10.1177/096228029600500305
19. Hamorsky KT, Bushau-Sprinkle AM, Kitterman K, et al. Serological assessment of SARS-CoV-2 infection during the first wave of the pandemic in Louisville Kentucky. *Sci Rep.* 2021;11(1):18285. https://doi.org/10.1038/s41598-021-97423-z
20. Sempos CT, Tian L. Adjusting coronavirus prevalence estimates for laboratory test kit error. *Am J Epidemiol.* 2021;190(1):109–115. https://doi.org/10.1093/aje/kwaa174
21. Alfego D, Sullivan A, Poirier B, et al. A population-based analysis of the longevity of SARS-CoV-2 antibody seropositivity in the United States. *EClinicalMedicine.* 2021;36:100902. https://doi.org/10.1016/j.eclinm.2021.100902
22. Harris PA, Taylor R, Thielke R, Payne J, Gonzalez N, Conde JG. Research Electronic Data Capture (REDCap)—a metadata-driven methodology and workflow process for providing translational research informatics support. *J Biomed Inform.* 2009;42(2):377–381. https://doi.org/10.1016/j.jbi.2008.08.010
23. Harris PA, Taylor R, Minor BL, et al. The REDCap consortium. Building an international community of software platform partners. *J Biomed Inform.* 2019;95:103208. https://doi.org/10.1016/j.jbi.2019.103208
24. Smith T, Holm RH, Keith RJ, et al. Quantifying the relationship between sub-population wastewater samples and community-wide SARS-CoV-2 seroprevalence. *Sci Total Environ.* 2022;853:158567. https://doi.org/10.1016/j.scitotenv.2022.158567
25. Shapiro MF, Berk ML, Berry SH, et al. National probability samples in studies of low-prevalence diseases. Part I: Perspectives and lessons from the HIV cost and services utilization study. *Health Serv Res.* 1999;34(5 pt 1):951–968.
26. Yu H, Yang CC, Yu P, Liu K. Emotion diffusion effect: negative sentiment COVID-19 tweets of public organizations attract more responses from followers. *PLoS One.* 2022;17(3):e0264794. https://doi.org/10.1371/journal.pone.0264794
27. Paulose-Ram R, Graber JE, Woodwell D, Ahluwalia N. The National Health and Nutrition Examination Survey (NHANES), 2021–2022: adapting data collection in a COVID-19 environment. *Am J Public Health.* 2021;111(12):2149–2156. https://doi.org/10.2105/AJPH.2021.306517
28. Hedlin D. Is there a "safe area" where the nonresponse rate has only a modest effect on bias despite non-ignorable nonresponse? *Int Stat Rev.* 2020;88(3):642–657. https://doi.org/10.1111/insr.12359
29. Hedt BL, Pagano M. Health indicators: eliminating bias from convenience sampling estimators. *Stat Med.* 2011;30(5):560–568. https://doi.org/10.1002/sim.3920
30. Tai DBG, Shah A, Doubeni CA, et al. The disproportionate impact of COVID-19 on racial and ethnic minorities in the United States. *Clin Infect Dis.* 2021;72(4):703–706. https://doi.org/10.1093/cid/ciaa815

Public Health Impacts of Vaccines for COVID-19 and Beyond: Opportunities to Overcome Technical and Regulatory Barriers for Randomized Trials

Lee Kennedy-Shaffer, PhD

The COVID-19 pandemic has revealed the importance of the population-scale effects of both diseases and interventions. Vaccines have had an enormous impact, greatly reducing the suffering caused by COVID-19. Clinical trials have focused on individual-level clinical benefits, however, so the broader effects of the vaccines on preventing infection and transmission, and their overall effect at the community level, remain unclear.

These questions can be addressed through alternative designs for vaccine trials, including assessing different endpoints and randomizing at the cluster instead of individual level. Although these designs exist, various factors have limited their use as preauthorization pivotal trials. They face statistical, epidemiological, and logistical limitations as well as regulatory barriers and uncertainty.

Addressing these hindrances through research, communication, and policy can improve the evidence base of vaccines, their strategic deployment, and population health, both in the COVID-19 pandemic and in future infectious disease outbreaks. (*Am J Public Health*. 2023;113(7):778–785. https://doi.org/10.2105/AJPH.2023.307302)

AJPH July 2023, Vol 113, No. 7

Three years into the COVID-19 pandemic, its effects are still being felt by individuals every day, and they will continue to be studied for years to come. The impacts have been wide ranging, affecting not just physical health but mental health, economics, politics, and society more broadly. As various pharmaceutical and nonpharmaceutical interventions have been promoted, implemented, and rolled back, this pandemic has clarified the need for timely assessment of their effects. Thinking critically about relevant endpoints and effect measures will be key to scaling up effective solutions to future epidemics, as well as continuing the fight against COVID-19.

Preauthorization clinical trials have been the primary tool to assess the effects of the COVID-19 vaccines. These randomized controlled trials (RCTs), with results published beginning in late 2020 and early 2021, were designed to assess vaccine safety and efficacy against symptomatic COVID-19.[1] The results were overwhelmingly positive, with several vaccines reporting estimates of vaccine efficacy above 60%[2,3] and at least 3 reporting estimates above 90%,[4] leading to rapid authorization and deployment. In addition, many trials included severe COVID-19 as a secondary endpoint and demonstrated efficacy there as well.[1–4] In individually randomizing large numbers of participants and focusing on symptomatic and severe COVID-19 as outcomes, these trials responded to US Food and Drug Administration (FDA) guidance issued in June 2020.[5] The development and deployment of the vaccines with unprecedented speed has prevented millions of hospitalizations and deaths in the United States and more abroad.[6]

Although these early studies and those that followed on other vaccine candidates certainly justified the authorization and use of these vaccines, they left several key public health questions unanswered. Among them are the effects that deployment of the vaccine on a wide scale would have on the population-level burden of severe acute respiratory syndrome coronavirus 2 (SARS-CoV-2) infection and COVID-19 disease. Because the RCTs that were conducted randomized individuals and measured symptomatic disease as the primary endpoint, they could not specifically estimate vaccine efficacy in terms of protecting against asymptomatic infection or onward transmission of the infection,[1] nor could they estimate the indirect and overall effects that vaccine deployment would have on those in the same community as a vaccinated individual without outcome measurements on those other individuals.[7]

News articles have highlighted these remaining questions in the context of government messaging and individual choices to take the vaccine as well as the push for new versions of the vaccine.[8,9] Although more recent observational and biological evidence indicates effectiveness beyond just symptomatic disease, more reliable estimates of the overall effects are lacking, leading to unclear messaging and policy implications.[8] In an era of frequent outbreaks and epidemics, these questions will continue to arise as vaccine developers address the latest threats, including both new waves of current diseases and new emerging infections.

To determine the public health benefit of vaccines during outbreaks and to deploy and provide messaging on vaccines with the best available evidence, we need to reconsider the evidence requested by regulators and the questions answered by pivotal clinical trials. Here I describe the current predominant approach to pivotal vaccine trials and highlight 2 potential alternative trial designs—evaluating infection- and transmission-relevant endpoints and conducting cluster RCTs (cRCTs)—that can address these questions. These approaches do have limitations, drawbacks, and research challenges that differ from the current paradigm. Addressing these challenges to develop a population-focused approach to trials, however, can improve the public health evidence base and, in turn, enable better assessments of policy trade-offs and improve responses.

PIVOTAL VACCINE TRIALS

RCTs for drug approvals (specifically, phase III or "pivotal" clinical trials) need to balance several, often competing goals, including those involving technical demands (e.g., maximizing statistical power and identifying a meaningful estimand) and logistical demands (e.g., the ethics, recruitment, speed, and costs of the trial). It generally falls to the drug's sponsor, in consultation with national regulatory authorities, to make the key trial design decisions.[10] These decisions are shaped by national and international guidance, such as that the primary endpoint should "provid[e] the most clinically relevant and convincing evidence directly related to the primary objective of the trial."[11]

In the case of prelicensure (or, in the COVID-19 case, preauthorization) vaccine trials, the objective has often been demonstrating clinical benefits for the individual vaccine recipients. Most such trials have thus been individually randomized controlled trials that focused on direct protection, leaving broader assessments of vaccine effectiveness in communities for postapproval (so-called "phase IV") studies.[12] Generally, then, primary endpoints have been symptomatic or severe disease, depending on the frequency of outcomes needed to ensure adequate statistical power.[1]

For example, according to FDA guidance for COVID-19 vaccine trials in June 2020, "the most direct approach to demonstrate effectiveness . . . is based on clinical endpoint efficacy trials showing protection against disease."[5] Specifically, the guidance noted that laboratory-confirmed COVID-19 disease or SARS-CoV-2 infection would be an "acceptable primary endpoint" and that symptomatic, virologically confirmed infection and severe COVID-19 should be included as primary or secondary endpoints.[5] This guidance—and the choices made in early trials in response to it—shapes not only the initial evidence gathered but the endpoints used in later comparison studies and studies for correlates of protection.[5,13]

These trials, however, focused on only a subset of the breadth of effects vaccines can have on individuals and communities. By measuring different outcomes among trial participants, investigators can estimate different vaccine effects, such as the effect on susceptibility to infection, progression from infection to disease, or infectiousness.[14] By contrast, assessing community-level effects through cRCTs enables assessment of vaccine effectiveness at a higher level, capturing both the direct effects of the vaccine on the vaccinated individual and the indirect protection conferred to nearby individuals.[15]

Because of the standard expectations for phase III trials, specific regulatory guidance, and the designs chosen in the case of COVID-19, assessment of these alternative effects has largely been left to postauthorization studies.[16] These studies can provide important evidence for the public and policymakers.[8] However, they are often observational studies, which may suffer from biases and reflect changing epidemic conditions.[4,7,16] These issues can be obviated through cluster randomization, but cRCTs after vaccine authorization often face ethical or legal barriers to randomization.[12,17]

The value of answering these public health–relevant questions in early trials has been discussed for previous infectious disease outbreaks[18,19] as well as in the COVID-19 case.[1,7] Alternative designs proved valuable in assessing Ebola vaccine candidates in West Africa in the 2014 outbreak.[12] Identifying community benefits of vaccination and honestly acknowledging its limitations can build trust in the vaccine and potentially inspire uptake.[12,20] The extent of indirect protection also affects how health resources should be distributed, improves postvaccine modeling of the epidemic, allows cost–benefit decisions that fully account for public health benefits, and helps inform assessments of ongoing nonpharmaceutical interventions.[12,16,18,19] Looking forward, these properties should also inform the development and evaluation of boosters and next-generation vaccines.[9,20] Full assessment of vaccines thus requires a broader array of designs than have commonly been used for pivotal trials.

ALTERNATIVE ENDPOINTS FOR VACCINE TRIALS

Endpoints other than symptomatic disease can be used to assess vaccine efficacy against infection or transmission. If infection—regardless of symptoms—is used as an endpoint by testing all or a random sample of trial participants at some point in time, vaccine efficacy against viral positivity (i.e., a combination of acquisition and duration of infection) can be assessed.[21] If a proxy of transmissibility—for example, the secondary attack rate among a defined set of close contacts or a biological proxy of infectiousness—can be identified and tested in that sample, vaccine efficacy against transmission can also be estimated.[22,23]

Two of the pivotal vaccine trials did assess efficacy against infection through either regular virologic testing or serologic testing after some time had passed, providing early evidence of vaccine efficacy against infection.[16] The ChAdOx1 vaccine study included weekly swabbing for a secondary analysis and revealed a significant effect against positivity, albeit lower than the measured effect against symptomatic disease.[2] A later analysis also showed a reduced viral load among vaccinated individuals in a subset of tested individuals who had such data.[24] The Ad26.COV2.S study used serologic testing after 71 days to identify participants who had been infected after randomization and revealed efficacy similar to that associated with symptomatic disease.[3]

Although these secondary endpoints were valuable, they involved smaller sample sizes than the primary endpoint and only scratched the surface of broader effects that could be estimated. Observational studies provided evidence that vaccines reduced transmissibility as well by both identifying reductions in onward transmission among, for example, household members[25] or other close contacts[26] and by measuring proxies such as the polymerase chain reaction cycle threshold (related to the viral load),[27] viral culture viability,[28] and rapid antigen test positivity.[29]

Despite the value of this observational evidence, these studies suffer from limitations. As with all observational studies, the risk of unmeasured confounding and selection bias could have biased the results.[16] Specifically, comparing secondary attack rates depends on index case identification, and detecting onward transmission accurately and in a timely way[30] and comparing viral loads can involve substantial bias, especially without randomization or with time-varying risks.[22,31]

In addition, the delay inherent in these studies—which must be conducted after vaccine rollout—limits their usefulness in informing vaccine deployment policies and the need for concurrent nonpharmaceutical interventions. Prelicensure RCTs addressing these endpoints would provide crucial effect estimates more quickly and more reliably. In addition, they would provide a foundation for later studies of boosters, vaccine effectiveness waning, and next-generation vaccines by generating highly reliable evidence of the initial effectiveness of vaccines against transmission endpoints. That would allow changes over time to be measured directly (e.g., assessing waning over time through post-unblinding follow-up[32]) or assessed in new studies (e.g., assessments of effectiveness against new variants[33]) and compared with initial findings, which would inform public health priorities and policies.

CLUSTER RANDOMIZATION AND OVERALL EFFECTIVENESS

Another method to understand a vaccine's impact on a population is a cRCT, which provides investigators with evidence on the community impact of an intervention. Instead of allocating individuals to either the control or vaccine arm, cRCTs allocate clusters of individuals; these clusters can be households, contacts of an index individual, schools, workplaces, or geographic units.[4,34] Individuals within clusters may or may not be required to take the vaccine, and thus cRCTs often reflect deployment in practice and are used to investigate the effects of postlicensure policies or strategies.[34] Through the clustering, cRCTs allow investigators to measure the overall effectiveness at the cluster level, accounting for both direct and indirect benefits to all individuals in the cluster.[15,18] If there are indirect effects of the vaccine (e.g., preventing infections or reducing infectiousness), the overall effect—and the total effect on vaccinated individuals specifically—will be larger than the direct vaccine efficacy.

Various types of cRCTs have been proposed or used to measure the effectiveness of nonvaccine interventions in the COVID-19 pandemic and vaccines in previous infectious disease outbreaks. Masks and hydroxychloroquine, among other interventions, were tested through cRCTs clustered by village and close contacts of an infected individual, respectively.[35,36] Vaccines designed primarily to work by blocking transmission, such as a recent malaria vaccine candidate, are particularly good candidates for cRCTs.[37]

In the 2014 Ebola outbreak, several cRCT designs were considered to test vaccines.[38] A ring design that randomized contacts (and contacts of contacts) of infected individuals—as a cluster—to the vaccine or control arm was used, demonstrating high effectiveness in preventing cases.[38] Even earlier, a subtype of cRCT known as a stepped-wedge cRCT was designed to assess a hepatitis B vaccine in The Gambia, with the vaccine rolled out to new geographic areas in phases.[39] This design has advantages, especially when supplies or program staff are constrained, as well as specific disadvantages. By capturing indirect effects and allowing for ease of logistics via operationalization at the cluster level, cRCTs have proven useful in infectious disease settings.[38]

Relatedly, observational studies involving cluster-level policies (e.g., state-level vaccine mandates for hospital workers[40]) have shown that when mandates are possible, cluster-level analyses can demonstrate the effectiveness of certain interventions. Conducting cluster-level studies earlier, when randomization is still ethical and feasible, would reduce the risk of bias in these analyses.[38] In this way, cRCTs can be useful tools to measure both the effectiveness of policies (e.g., availability or promotion of vaccines) and, in settings where uptake will be high as a result of mandates or high prelicensure desirability, the effectiveness of widespread vaccination itself.

TRADE-OFFS, LIMITATIONS, AND RESEARCH DEMANDS

Although they provide valuable public health information, these alternative vaccine trial designs have drawbacks and limitations as well. They also provide opportunities for research to address these limitations, quantify the trade-offs between competing designs, and address regulatory uncertainty. Box 1 summarizes these designs and estimands as well as some of the challenges they pose.[2,3,12,15,18,19,21–29,30,34–39,41–44]

These approaches often require more complex statistical modeling, demand stronger epidemiological assumptions, or face reduced power relative to standard approaches. Measuring transmission directly among close contacts requires a clear and consistent definition of those contacts; either the trial participants must be tested regularly, with additional testing for contacts of infected participants, or only contacts of symptomatic participants are tested, which may lead to a biased estimate if the vaccine effect on symptomatic infection is different from its effect on asymptomatic infections.[30] Moreover, these approaches are limited to identifying transmission among a defined type of contact, ignoring other pathways for transmission, and modeling of other infection sources is often needed to improve validity and precision.[25,26]

Estimating vaccine efficacy against transmission via a proxy for infectiousness will either face limited power at a single point in time or require a more complex model to accommodate repeated sampling.[22,23] Initially, a suitable proxy must be found that both is easy enough to sample on a wide scale and has a known relationship to transmission. Then numerous assumptions must be made about the proxy, including that its relationship with infectiousness is not affected by vaccination.[22] Although, for example, polymerase chain reaction cycle threshold values and rapid antigen test positivity rates both may be reasonable proxies for COVID-19 transmissibility, this may not hold true for future variants or other infections.[41] Viral culture positivity, a common indicator of transmissibility, is more expensive, time consuming, and laborious to determine and requires a specialized laboratory, generally resulting in a smaller sample size or higher costs.[28,29] To use these designs, research into a suitable proxy must be prioritized early in the outbreak.

Regulators also need to ensure appropriate consideration of these endpoints, possibly by allowing alternative specifications of validation and sensitivity to meet population, rather than individual, considerations.[5] Uncertainty about these proxy measures and their relationship to actual transmission events is a major barrier to and limitation of such studies.

BOX 1— Selected Alternative Designs for Randomized Vaccine Trials and Their Potential Challenges

Primary Endpoint/ Design	Estimand	Potential Challenges	Selected References
Individually randomized controlled trials			
Virologic test positivity	Vaccine efficacy against prevalent infection	Reduced power or requires frequent testing and modeling	Methodology[21,23]; RCT example[2]
Serologic test positivity	Vaccine efficacy against incident infection	Vaccination may affect test performance; cannot identify or analyze time to infection; may lead to smaller sample sizes	RCT example[3]; observational example[35]
Secondary attack rate in defined contacts	Vaccine efficacy against infectiousness given infection	Requires large amount of testing; risk of bias in index case and contact identification; limited generalizability to other contacts	Methodology[30]; observational examples[25,26]
Virologic test cycle threshold value	Vaccine efficacy against transmission	More costly; requires assumptions/model of transmissibility and justified proxy	Methodology[22,23]; RCT example[24]; observational example[27]; biological justification[41]
Rapid antigen test positivity	Vaccine efficacy against transmission	Requires validated test properties for at-home use	Observational example[29]; biological justification[41]
Viral culture positivity	Vaccine efficacy against transmission	More costly; requires appropriate laboratory; requires assumptions/model of transmissibility	Observational example[28]; biological justification[41]
Cluster randomized controlled trials			
Parallel-arm cRCT	Overall or total vaccine effectiveness at the clustering level	Group consent ethics; large simultaneous rollout; estimand value depends on clustering level and outbreak trajectory	Methodology[34,42]; RCT examples[19,35–37]; discussion[15,18,19,38,43]
Ring design cRCT	Overall or total vaccine effectiveness for contacts (or larger rings)	Estimand corresponds to specific vaccine rollout strategy	RCT example[36]; discussion[12,38]
Stepped-wedge cRCT	Depends on analysis method	Slower, reduced power, dependent on analysis method	Methodology[44]; RCT example[39]; discussion[38,43]

Note. cRCT = cluster randomized controlled trial; RCT = randomized controlled trial.

Often randomizing a relatively small number of clusters, cRCTs can face the risk of imbalance between arms, and the correlation between participants leads to less precise effect estimates.[34] Although the larger overall effect size being estimated in a cRCT could in theory lead to greater statistical power than a comparably sized individually randomized trial, this is rarely the case in practical settings.[42] The reduction in power is even more pronounced for stepped-wedge cRCTs, which also face potential biases under standard analysis methods.[44] There is recent and ongoing research into improving the efficiency of analysis methods and the validity of designs for cRCTs, as well as tools that quantify the inherent trade-offs.[43] Specific research on the high temporal sensitivity of cluster-level outcomes would be particularly valuable, especially if designers can use it to consider how simultaneous interventions that “flatten the curve” influence the measured effects.

Generalizability and interpretation of the measured effects also pose a challenge for these designs. Effects on the likelihood of onward transmission may change as pathogens evolve and behavior changes.[1,9] The indirect effects that are measured in cRCTs depend on many factors: uptake of the vaccine within the clusters, the reproduction number of the infection, the number of susceptible individuals in the population, and other preventive measures taken.[15,42] This can result in overall vaccine effectiveness estimates that are specific to the context of the trial and may be less generalizable to other locations or time points.

For example, although cRCTs may randomize clusters to availability or promotion of vaccines, this may not ensure that all individuals within treated clusters receive the vaccines and that no individuals within control clusters do. The vaccine effectiveness estimands targeted in these trials, then, more accurately capture the effects of the policy (e.g., of availability, promotion, or mandate) than vaccine efficacy itself.[18,34] Although direct vaccine efficacy estimates from individually randomized trials may also not be fully generalizable (e.g., this depends on the pathogen strain mix at a given location and time point,[9] as we have seen with

SARS-CoV-2), this is likely a greater challenge for cRCTs.[18] Research on the time dependence of these effects, and whether accurate predictions can be made when generalizing to other populations and time points, could alleviate some of these concerns.

In addition, research on how best to communicate such results, as well as which types of evidence are most convincing to the public, would be valuable. Messaging around vaccines has been challenging because of differing notions of the primary purpose of the COVID-19 vaccines.[20] A fuller understanding of their effects, coupled with effective communication strategies, could improve that.

Logistically, trials must balance speed, cost, and recruitment ability. Routine testing of a large number of trial participants (and potentially their contacts) is expensive and potentially logistically difficult.[38] The use of rapid or at-home tests introduces more human variability and the potential for reduced sensitivity or specificity. Serologic tests for any past infection reduce the need for frequent testing but require the assumption that seroconversion does not differ between vaccinated and unvaccinated individuals, which may not be true in all settings.[45] They also limit the ability to assess time to infection, which can bias comparisons and limit public health understanding of interventions that delay infections.[44] Moreover, the use of serologic tests may limit sample sizes; 2 large-scale trials saw drastically limited sample sizes for their serologic test outcomes.[3,35] Stepped-wedge cRCTs can be attractive when resources are limited (and would be rolled out in a staggered fashion in any event) but may be slower than other designs.[38] As with RCTs in general, all of these designs face trade-offs among their numerous goals and constraints.

Phase III trials must also collect safety data and adhere to ethical standards of consent and monitoring. Although changing the primary endpoint need not remove any safety endpoints, some safety endpoints may fit better among certain designs (e.g., serologic testing and serum-based lab safety endpoints). Safety and monitoring in cRCTs can be more complex but can be achieved through passive surveillance with appropriate follow-up length.[37] Decisions surrounding consent for randomization are often challenging for cRCTs, and many are conducted as open-label postlicensure trials, risking bias and limiting their ability to inform authorization and rollout.[17,34]

Research and tools to quantify these trade-offs (e.g., see the tool developed by Bellan et al.[43]) may prove useful to investigators balancing these competing concerns. Also, broader planning and discussion of ethical and logistical issues (e.g., as described by Wilder-Smith et al.,[12] Delrieu et al.,[37] and Dean et al.[38]) can address these concerns without the time pressure of a public health emergency. Financial support for larger trials, if needed to gain broader information on effects, could persuade sponsors to be more ambitious in trial design as well.

Finally, historical and contemporary reliance on individual RCTs with clinically focused endpoints for pivotal vaccine trials—along with specific guidance recommending those types of trials—has left uncertainty about what evidence would be acceptable to national regulators and international bodies. For example, according to the FDA guidance for COVID-19 vaccine trials in June 2020, cRCTs "may be acceptable but require careful consideration of potential biases that are usually avoided with individual randomization."[5] Although this does not preclude cRCTs outright, it may leave sponsors uncertain about whether they are truly a viable pathway.

The recent focus in international regulatory guidance on choosing appropriate estimands should encourage a broader reconsideration of these alternative designs. The International Conference on Harmonisation, which lays out clinical trial principles that are adopted by many national regulatory agencies, put forward an addendum specifically focused on estimands.[46] This has led to a push for larger conversations about the most appropriate estimands, including endpoints and the compared populations, and more comprehensive reporting of these choices in statistical analysis plans.[47]

This is an opportunity to reevaluate the regulatory regime and ensure that designs most relevant for public health can be used in pivotal vaccine trials and in studies of correlates of protection. The European Medicines Agency has already indicated a willingness to authorize vaccines on the basis of population impacts, and the FDA has pathways that could be used to follow suit.[19] As decisions regarding acceptable clinical trial design occur mostly through guidance documents and conversations with regulators,[10] active guidance surrounding these possibilities from regulators and clarity for industry sponsors of trials will be necessary to move the needle.[17] Specific guidance on what data and justifications are needed for cRCTs or trials with nonclinical endpoints should be laid out for next-generation COVID-19 vaccine trials (including noninferiority trials) and considered for future outbreaks.

CONCLUSION

The COVID-19 pandemic has reinforced the importance of public health and considering effects on a population scale, which should encourage further discussion in the research community of the most appropriate study designs to answer crucial questions. Although the authorized vaccines have greatly reduced the toll of this epidemic, much is still unknown or only recently coming to light about their impact at the population level. These questions will only deepen as choices are made about deploying updated vaccines and the need for additional interventions as the disease continues to spread.[8,9] Although we have tools to evaluate these effects, their usefulness is limited after the initial trials and deployment.

Understanding the effect of vaccines on infections and transmission, not just disease, can inform an effective vaccine response to an outbreak and improve modeling of the epidemic and decision making surrounding concurrent public health measures.[12,16,19] These issues can be understood in time for incorporation into vaccine planning through careful consideration of vaccine trial designs. Choosing an endpoint through the lens of public health (e.g., prevalent infection or a proxy for transmission) can provide an important estimate of vaccine effectiveness. In addition, randomizing at an appropriate scale via a cRCT can provide insight into the vaccine's indirect and overall effectiveness. These choices are not without drawbacks, and research into appropriate endpoints and methods, and into the trade-offs they entail, is necessary to ensure reliability and inform trial design selection.

Moreover, this will require a change in focus at the regulatory and policymaking levels. Trial sponsors need to be allowed, encouraged, and incentivized to conduct such trials with a public health outcome in mind. Regulators will need to update guidance and provide certainty about the role these trials can play. Finally, policymakers need to show a willingness to use the information provided by these trials to shape public health policy. By facing these challenges, we can embrace the opportunity to improve public health in the ongoing COVID-19 pandemic and use what we have learned from the COVID-19 vaccine experience to improve public health in future outbreaks. AJPH

ABOUT THE AUTHOR

The author is with the Department of Mathematics and Statistics, Vassar College, Poughkeepsie, NY.

CORRESPONDENCE

Correspondence should be sent to Lee Kennedy-Shaffer, PhD, Box 226, Vassar College, 124 Raymond Ave, Poughkeepsie, NY 12604-0226 (e-mail: lkennedyshaffer@vassar.edu). Reprints can be ordered at http://www.ajph.org by clicking the "Reprints" link.

PUBLICATION INFORMATION

Full Citation: Kennedy-Shaffer L. Public health impacts of vaccines for COVID-19 and beyond: opportunities to overcome technical and regulatory barriers for randomized trials. *Am J Public Health*. 2023;113(7):778–785.

Acceptance Date: March 20, 2023.

DOI: https://doi.org/10.2105/AJPH.2023.307302

ACKNOWLEDGMENTS

I thank the reviewers and editors for their helpful suggestions.

CONFLICTS OF INTEREST

The author has no conflicts of interest to disclose.

HUMAN PARTICIPANT PROTECTION

This work did not involve original research including any human participants.

REFERENCES

1. Mehrotra DV, Janes HE, Fleming TR, et al. Clinical endpoints for evaluating efficacy in COVID-19 vaccine trials. *Ann Intern Med*. 2021;174(2):221–228. https://doi.org/10.7326/M20-6169
2. Voysey M, Clemens SAC, Madhi SA, et al. Safety and efficacy of the ChAdOx1 nCoV-19 vaccine (AZD1222) against SARS-CoV-2: an interim analysis of four randomised controlled trials in Brazil, South Africa, and the UK. *Lancet*. 2021;397(10269):99–111. https://doi.org/10.1016/S0140-6736(20)32661-1
3. Sadoff J, Gray G, Vandebosch A, et al. Safety and efficacy of single-dose Ad26.COV2.S vaccine against Covid-19. *N Engl J Med*. 2021;384(23):2187–2201. https://doi.org/10.1056/NEJMoa2101544
4. Kim JH, Marks F, Clemens JD. Looking beyond COVID-19 vaccine phase 3 trials. *Nat Med*. 2021;27(2):205–211. https://doi.org/10.1038/s41591-021-01230-y
5. US Food and Drug Administration, Center for Biologics Evaluation and Research. Development and licensure of vaccines to prevent COVID-19: guidance for industry. Available at: https://www.fda.gov/media/139638/download. Accessed March 15, 2023.
6. Fitzpatrick MC, Moghadas SM, Pandey A, Galvani AP. Two years of US COVID-19 vaccines have prevented millions of deaths and hospitalizations. Available at: https://www.commonwealthfund.org/blog/2022/two-years-covid-vaccines-prevented-millions-deaths-hospitalizations. Accessed December 20, 2022.
7. Lipsitch M, Dean NE. Understanding COVID-19 vaccine efficacy. *Science*. 2020;370(6518):763–765. https://doi.org/10.1126/science.abe5938
8. Mallapaty S. Can COVID vaccines stop transmission? Scientists race to find answers. *Nature*. 2021 [Epub ahead of print]. https://doi.org/10.1038/d41586-021-00450-z
9. Cohen J. Making broader coronavirus vaccines is a struggle. *Science*. 2022;377(6606):566–567. https://doi.org/10.1126/science.ade2363
10. Darrow JJ. Pharmaceutical efficacy: the illusory legal standard. *Wash Lee Law Rev*. 2013;70(4):2073–2136.
11. International Conference on Harmonisation. E9: statistical principles for clinical trials. Available at: https://ich.org/page/efficacy-guidelines. Accessed December 22, 2022.
12. Wilder-Smith A, Longini I, Zuber PL, et al. The public health value of vaccines beyond efficacy: methods, measures and outcomes. *BMC Med*. 2017;15(1):138. https://doi.org/10.1186/s12916-017-0911-8
13. Gilbert PB, Donis RO, Koup RA, Fong Y, Plotkin SA, Follmann DA. Covid-19 milestone attained—a correlate of protection for vaccines. *N Engl J Med*. 2022;387(24):2203–2206. https://doi.org/10.1056/NEJMp2211314
14. Halloran ME, Longini IM, Struchiner CJ. Design and interpretation of vaccine field studies. *Epidemiol Rev*. 1999;21(1):73–88. https://doi.org/10.1093/oxfordjournals.epirev.a017990
15. Halloran ME, Struchiner CJ. Study designs for dependent happenings. *Epidemiology*. 1991;2(5):331–338. https://doi.org/10.1097/00001648-199109000-00004
16. Richterman A, Meyerowitz EA, Cevik M. Indirect protection by reducing transmission: ending the pandemic with severe acute respiratory syndrome coronavirus 2 vaccination. *Open Forum Infect Dis*. 2022;9(2):ofab259. https://doi.org/10.1093/ofid/ofab259
17. Copas A, Murray DM, Roberts JN. Thirteenth annual UPenn conference on statistical issues in

clinical trials: cluster-randomized clinical trials—opportunities and challenges. *Clin Trials.* 2022; 19(4):422–431. https://doi.org/10.1177/17407745221101284

18. Clemens J. Evaluating new vaccines for developing countries. Efficacy or effectiveness? *JAMA.* 1996;275(5):390–397. https://doi.org/10.1001/jama.1996.03530290060038
19. Saadatian-Elahi M, Horstick O, Breiman RF, et al. Beyond efficacy: the full public health impact of vaccines. *Vaccine.* 2016;34(9):1139–1147. https://doi.org/10.1016/j.vaccine.2016.01.021
20. Schraer R. COVID jab probably does protect those around you. Available at: https://www.bbc.com/news/health-56514470. Accessed November 21, 2022.
21. Lipsitch M, Kahn R. Interpreting vaccine efficacy trial results for infection and transmission. *Vaccine.* 2021;39(30):4082–4088. https://doi.org/10.1016/j.vaccine.2021.06.011
22. Kennedy-Shaffer L, Kahn R, Lipsitch M. Estimating vaccine efficacy against transmission via effect on viral load. *Epidemiology.* 2021;32(6):820–828. https://doi.org/10.1097/EDE.0000000000001415
23. Follmann DA, Fay MP. Vaccine efficacy at a point in time. *Biostatistics.* 2022 [Epub ahead of print]. https://doi.org/10.1093/biostatistics/kxac008
24. Emary KRW, Golubchik T, Aley PK, et al. Efficacy of ChAdOx1 nCoV-19 (AZD1222) vaccine against SARS-CoV-2 variant of concern 202012/01 (B.1.1.7): an exploratory analysis of a randomised controlled trial. *Lancet.* 2021;397(10282):1351–1362. https://doi.org/10.1016/S0140-6736(21)00628-0
25. Prunas O, Warren JL, Crawford FW, et al. Vaccination with BNT162b2 reduces transmission of SARS-CoV-2 to household contacts in Israel. *Science.* 2022;375(6585):1151–1154. https://doi.org/10.1126/science.abl4292
26. Tan ST, Kwan AT, Rodríguez-Barraquer I, et al. Infectiousness of SARS-CoV-2 breakthrough infections and reinfections during the Omicron wave. *Nat Med.* 2023;29(2):358–365. https://doi.org/10.1038/s41591-022-02138-x
27. Levine-Tiefenbrun M, Yelin I, Katz R, et al. Initial report of decreased SARS-CoV-2 viral load after inoculation with the BNT162b2 vaccine. *Nat Med.* 2021;27(5):790–792. https://doi.org/10.1038/s41591-021-01316-7
28. HEROES-RECOVER Network. Association of mRNA vaccination with clinical and virologic features of COVID-19 among US essential and frontline workers. *JAMA.* 2022;328(15):1523–1533. https://doi.org/10.1001/jama.2022.18550
29. Regev-Yochay G, Amit S, Bergwerk M, et al. Decreased infectivity following BNT162b2 vaccination: a prospective cohort study in Israel. *Lancet Reg Health Eur.* 2021;7:100150. https://doi.org/10.1016/j.lanepe.2021.100150
30. Accorsi EK, Qiu X, Rumpler E, et al. How to detect and reduce potential sources of biases in studies of SARS-CoV-2 and COVID-19. *Eur J Epidemiol.* 2021; 36(2):179–196. https://doi.org/10.1007/s10654-021-00727-7
31. Hay JA, Kennedy-Shaffer L, Kanjilal S, et al. Estimating epidemiologic dynamics from cross-sectional viral load distributions. *Science.* 2021;373(6552): eabh0635. https://doi.org/10.1126/science.abh0635
32. Baden LR, Sahly HME, Essink B, et al. Phase 3 trial of mRNA-1273 during the Delta-variant surge. *N Engl J Med.* 2021;385(26):2485–2487. https://doi.org/10.1056/NEJMc2115597
33. Eyre DW, Taylor D, Purver M, et al. Effect of COVID-19 vaccination on transmission of Alpha and Delta variants. *N Engl J Med.* 2022;386(8):744–756. https://doi.org/10.1056/NEJMoa2116597
34. Hayes RJ, Moulton LH. *Cluster Randomised Trials.* 2nd ed. Boca Raton, FL: Chapman and Hall/CRC; 2017.
35. Abaluck J, Kwong LH, Styczynski A, et al. Impact of community masking on COVID-19: a cluster-randomized trial in Bangladesh. *Science.* 2022; 375(6577):eabi9069. https://doi.org/10.1126/science.abi9069
36. Mitjà O, Corbacho-Monné M, Ubals M, et al. A cluster-randomized trial of hydroxychloroquine for prevention of COVID-19. *N Engl J Med.* 2021; 384(5):417–427. https://doi.org/10.1056/NEJMoa2021801
37. Delrieu I, Leboulleux D, Ivinson K, et al. Design of a phase III cluster randomized trial to assess the efficacy and safety of a malaria transmission blocking vaccine. *Vaccine.* 2015;33(13):1518–1526. https://doi.org/10.1016/j.vaccine.2015.01.050
38. Dean NE, Gsell PS, Brookmeyer R, et al. Design of vaccine efficacy trials during public health emergencies. *Sci Transl Med.* 2019;11(499):eaat0360. https://doi.org/10.1126/scitranslmed.aat0360
39. Gambia Hepatitis Study Group. The Gambia hepatitis intervention study. *Cancer Res.* 1987;47: 5782–5787.
40. Carrera M, Lawler EC, White C. Population mortality and laws encouraging influenza vaccination for hospital workers. *Ann Intern Med.* 2021;174(4): 444–452. https://doi.org/10.7326/M20-0413
41. Lee LYW, Rozmanowski S, Pang M, et al. Severe acute respiratory syndrome coronavirus 2 (SARS-CoV-2) infectivity by viral load, S gene variants and demographic factors, and the utility of lateral flow devices to prevent transmission. *Clin Infect Dis.* 2022;74(3):407–415. https://doi.org/10.1093/cid/ciab421
42. Hitchings MDT, Lipsitch M, Wang R, Bellan SE. Competing effects of indirect protection and clustering on the power of cluster-randomized controlled vaccine trials. *Am J Epidemiol.* 2018;187(8):1763–1771. https://doi.org/10.1093/aje/kwy047
43. Bellan SE, Eggo RM, Gsell PS, et al. An online decision tree for vaccine efficacy trial design during infectious disease epidemics: the InterVax-Tool. *Vaccine.* 2019;37(31):4376–4381. https://doi.org/10.1016/j.vaccine.2019.06.019
44. Kennedy-Shaffer L, Lipsitch M. Statistical properties of stepped wedge cluster-randomized trials in infectious disease outbreaks. *Am J Epidemiol.* 2020;189(11):1324–1332. https://doi.org/10.1093/aje/kwaa141
45. Follmann D, Janes HE, Buhule OD, et al. Antinucleocapsid antibodies after SARS-CoV-2 infection in the blinded phase of the randomized, placebo-controlled mRNA-1273 COVID-19 Vaccine Efficacy Clinical Trial. *Ann Intern Med.* 2022;175(9): 1258–1265. https://doi.org/10.7326/M22-1300
46. International Conference on Harmonisation. E9(R1): addendum on estimands and sensitivity analysis in clinical trials. Available at: https://ich.org/page/efficacy-guidelines. Accessed December 22, 2022.
47. Kang M, Kendall MA, Ribaudo H, et al. Incorporating estimands into clinical trial statistical analysis plans. *Clin Trials.* 2022;19(3):285–291. https://doi.org/10.1177/17407745221080463

Variation in End-of-Life Trajectories in Persons Aged 70 Years and Older, Sweden, 2018–2020

Marcus Ebeling, PhD, Anna C. Meyer, PhD, and Karin Modig, PhD

See also Feng, p. 716.

Objectives. To analyze variation in end-of-life trajectories with regard to elder care and medical care and how they relate to age, gender, and causes of death.

Methods. We analyzed all deaths of persons at age 70 years and older between the years 2018 and 2020 in Sweden, using a linkage of population registers. We applied latent class analysis to identify distinct types of end-of-life trajectories.

Results. We identified 6 different types of end-of-life trajectories. The types differed substantially in the amount of utilized elder care and medical care before death. Deaths characterized by high levels of elder care and medical care utilization become more common with age. The trajectory types show distinct cause-of-death profiles.

Conclusions. Most deaths today do not comply with what is often referred to as a "good" death (e.g., retaining control or requiring low levels of elder care). The results suggest that longer lifespans partly result from a prolonged dying process.

Public Health Implications. The current modes of dying call for a discussion about how we want to die in an era of increasing lifespans and aging societies. (*Am J Public Health*. 2023;113(7):786–794. https://doi.org/10.2105/AJPH.2023.307281)

AJPH July 2023, Vol 113, No. 7

An increasing number of people reach older ages, and, thus, many countries in the world are faced with increasing numbers of deaths every year. In Sweden, for instance, 25% more annual deaths are expected in 30 years.[1] The time before death is a critical and challenging period of life, and more deaths at higher ages may result in an increased burden on the health sector and on society at large. Insights are needed to fuel the debate about the value of death and dying in aging societies. Currently, we miss a comprehensive understanding of the variation in individual end-of-life trajectories and how deaths following a specific trajectory are distributed across genders, ages, and causes of death.

For many individuals, the end-of-life trajectory is characterized by the transition from becoming ill to death, which can take days or months for some and years for others. A sudden unexpected death compared with a death after a long and severe disease illustrates this in a simplified way. Continued medical progress has likely affected end-of-life trajectories by delaying the onset and improving survival for many diseases. This may have led to an extended period of disease accumulation and care needs at the end of life.

Few previous studies have aimed to identify commonalities across individual end-of-life trajectories. In 2 separate analyses, Lunney et al.[2,3] described 4 distinct trajectories based on physical functioning and medical care needs at the end of life. The pathway types include, for instance, terminal illness with a rapid decline in physical functioning, or frailty with a slow but continuous decline. Raab et al.[4] focused on joint patterns of physical and mental health. They identified 5 distinct trajectory types and found that functional limitations can go along with both a constantly high or low prevalence of depression symptoms at the end of life. A Finnish study described end-of-life care by predefining 4 different care profiles based on the primary place of residence and the care transitions during the last 6 months of life,[5] and a study of deaths in Ontario used the cause of death as grouping criteria.[6] Although all studies provided seminal insights into several different aspects of end-of-life trajectories, they either focused on a specific aspect, such as number or timing of care transitions, or they relied on a subsample of the population. End-of-life trajectories, therefore, were not linked to the societal level or analyzed in the context of total population mortality.

Analyses of population-level mortality are often centered around age, gender, and causes of death, and end-of-life trajectories are neglected. By incorporating how individuals move toward death, we will be able to draw a realistic picture about dying in an era of continuous health improvements and improve our understanding of the current and future challenges around the end of life in aging populations. For this, it is important to capture the full spectrum of end-of-life trajectories, including individuals who are traditionally hard to reach, such as individuals in long-term institutionalized care settings. In this study, we utilized high-resolution Swedish register data, which provided a unique opportunity to study end-of-life trajectories based on a complete enumeration of annual deaths.

Two characteristics are essential when studying end-of life trajectories: (1) When does the transition to death start? and (2) What constitutes the transition to death? The question of when does the pathway to death start, or, in other words, when do we start dying, is an essential question of life. Any answer will be incomplete, but attempting to find an answer is important—for instance, when it comes to deciding if a curative or a palliative treatment strategy is most suitable for a (terminally ill) patient. In this study, end-of-life trajectories are measured across the last year of life with a focus on elder care and medical care, 2 of the most relevant public health dimensions. Elder care in Sweden is publicly funded and assigned on the basis of individual needs. As a first choice, individuals are offered home care, and it is only when care needs can no longer be met at home that individuals are allowed to move into a care home.[7] This makes elder care status a suitable proxy for the degree of dependency at the end of life. Medical care utilization will be indicated by type and quantity of medical care, which are 2 important dimensions of end-of-life health care and health care expenditures, which are reportedly highest during the period before death.[8–10]

The aim of this study was to derive a classification of end-of-life trajectories and to investigate how they are distributed over age, gender, and causes of death. This will allow us to link the end of life to population mortality and shed more light on the overarching question: how do we die?

METHODS

The study included all deaths at age 70 years or older that occurred in Sweden between 2018 and 2020.

Data

We derived information on date and cause of death from the Cause of Death Register.[11] We extracted in- and outpatient care utilization during the last 12 months of life from the National Patient Register.[12,13] We assessed the quantity of medical care utilization as the number of days spent in a hospital for inpatient care and as the number of visits for outpatient care.

In addition, we considered the type of medical care, which we measured through the identifier of the field of medical activity (MVO). The MVO code indicates the type of clinic, or health center that provided medical care and is assigned to each record in the National Patient Register. We used this information to measure whether a person received acute care at least once (e.g., emergency care) and whether a person received some form of specialized clinical care (e.g., palliative care or home health care). Both are main pillars of end-of-life care.[14,15] Several different MVO codes were used to identify the 2 types of care (Table A, available as a supplement to the online version of this article at https://ajph.org).

We measured elder care by using the Social Service Register, which contains monthly information on publicly funded elder care.[7] Care status was measured 1 year before death and at death, distinguishing between 3 states: (1) no publicly funded elder care during the month, (2) any amount of home care indicated by a granted home care claim, and (3) living in an elder care home. Reliable information on elder care status was missing for less than 1% of deaths; we omitted these from the analysis. All data were available until December 31, 2020.

Analytical Strategy

We used latent class analysis (LCA) to identify common patterns of end-of-life trajectories across individuals. LCA is a statistical procedure to uncover homogeneous subgroups (latent classes) within a population, which are identified on the basis of the similarity of individual response patterns across a set of indicator variables. The indicator variables used in our analysis captured various aspects of elder care and medical care utilization in the last year of life. As a consequence, the identified subgroups included individuals with similar care-oriented end-of-life trajectories. The fitting procedure of LCA has been described in detail elsewhere.[16]

We considered 6 different indicator variables:

1. elder care status (no care, receiving home care, and living in a care home) 1 year before death,
2. elder care status at death,
3. inpatient care utilization over the course of the last year of life,
4. outpatient care utilization over the course of the last year of life,
5. acute care over the course of the last year of life, and
6. specialized clinical care over the course of the last year of life.

We classified medical care utilization into 3 groups: low, medium, and high. We based the groups on the lower (≤ 2 days or ≤ 1 visits), mid (3–17 days or 2–5 visits), and upper (> 17 days or > 5 visits) terciles of the distribution of hospital days (inpatient care) and visits to outpatient care across all individuals. To measure whether individuals received acute health care and specialized clinical care (e.g., palliative care), we created 2 binary variables, which indicate if a person had at least 1 record with a relevant MVO code.

We conducted the LCA separately for each calendar year (2018, 2019, and 2020). In all years, the optimal number of latent classes was 6, which we identified using the Bayesian information criterion, the Akaike information criterion, and the meaningfulness and size of the derived classes. We also evaluated the prediction performance of the model using the average latent class probability. We found all diagonal probabilities to be well above the lower threshold of 0.8 and off-diagonal probabilities to have small values, which suggests that the identified groups were reasonably different from each other (Table C, available as a supplement to the online version of this article at https://ajph.org).[17] In a second step, we analyzed how the derived pathway types were distributed over gender, age, and cause of death. This analysis provided further support for the chosen specification of the LCA model.[17]

We performed the statistical analysis with R version 4.1.1 (R Foundation for Statistical Computing, Vienna, Austria), and the poLCA package in R (version 1.4.1). Codes and other materials can be obtained online (https://doi.org/10.17605/OSF.IO/TYN7J). For data access, an application must be filed.

RESULTS

The total number of deaths in Sweden at age 70 years and older was 75 151 in 2018, 72 683 in 2019, and 81 275 in 2020 (Table B, available as a supplement to the online version of this article at https://ajph.org). This constitutes around 80% of the total annual number of deaths in Sweden in the respective years. The increase of death counts in 2020 is a consequence of the COVID-19 pandemic.

Figure 1 illustrates the identified types of end-of-life trajectories. The first row shows the proportion of deaths that followed the specific trajectory, averaged across the 3 considered years. The most common type was "terminally ill" (26% of all deaths), while "sudden death" and "impaired" (both 11%) were the least common types. The color coding in the figure refers to the probability of having a specific outcome on the respective indicator variable (e.g., the probability of receiving acute care among deaths being classified as "terminally ill"). Note that, in many cases, the estimates marked as being below or above the thresholds of 0.33 and 0.66 are close to zero or 1. We refer to Table D (available as a supplement to the online version of this article at https://ajph.org) for detailed estimates and a more nuanced presentation.

The indicator variables can be divided into 2 broader ones—elder care and medical care. We found the elder care variables to be most important for grouping the trajectories. In fact, using only elder care as an indicator variable would create 3 rather than 6 trajectory types. The "dependent" and "impaired" trajectories showed higher shares of elder care utilization. We chose labels to reflect the health status, and, thus, "impaired" refers to home care because individuals are still able to live in their own home, while "dependent" refers to care home residents because individuals cannot manage to live at home anymore. The "sudden deaths" and" terminally ill" trajectories had a low probability of receiving elder care during the last year of life.

When we added medical care, the 3 broader types were divided into 6 trajectories. The differences in medical care utilization made the "sudden deaths" and "terminally ill" groups 2 distinct trajectories. "Sudden deaths" showed a low medical care utilization, and, thus, none of the indicator variables suggested the approaching death, which is the main reason for the labeling. The "terminally ill" type displayed high medical care utilization and a need for specialized clinical and acute care, which we interpreted as a sign for the rapid progression of a terminal illness. Medical care utilization also distinguished the "impaired severe

AJPH July 2023, Vol 113, No. 7

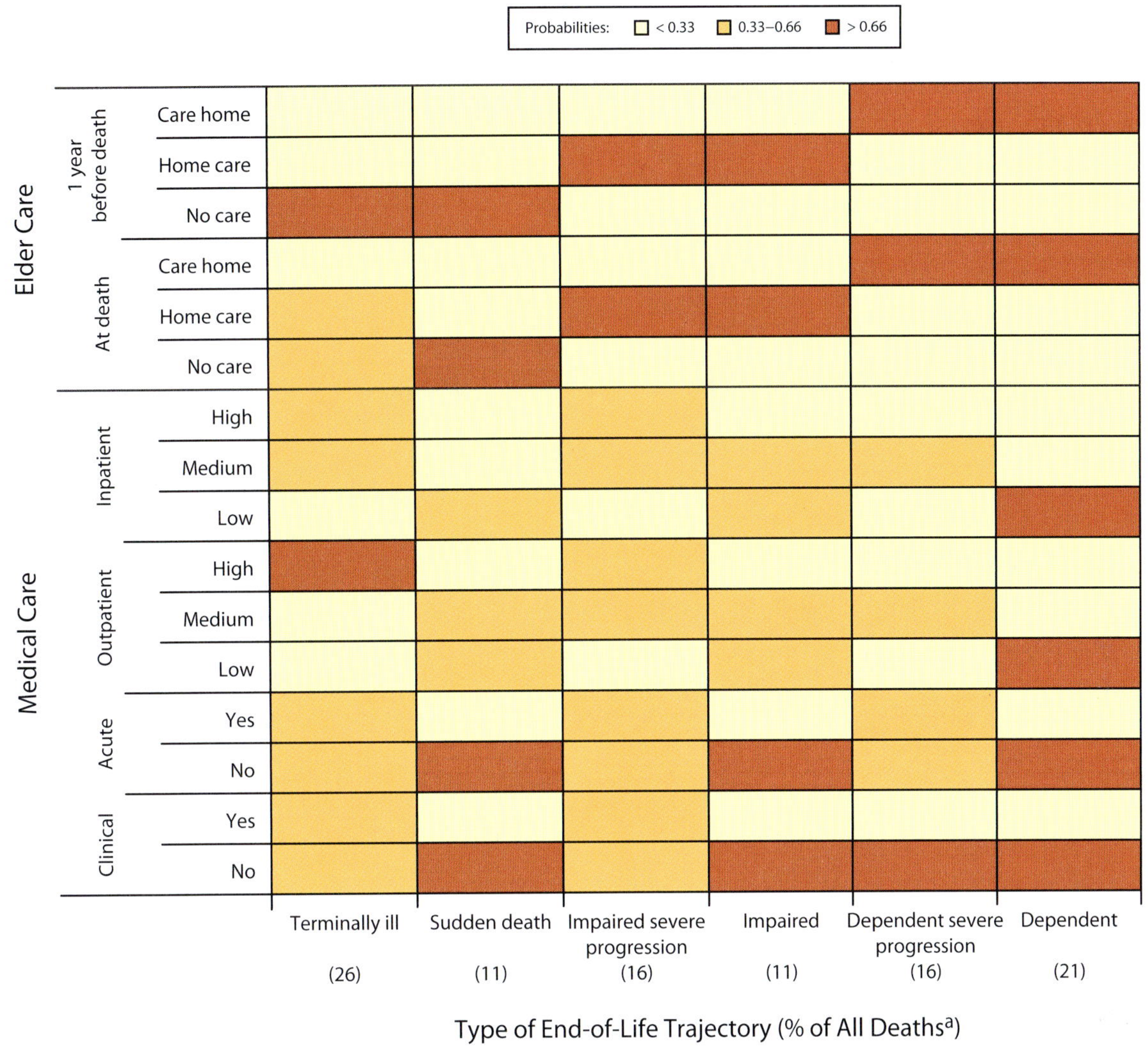

FIGURE 1— **End-of-Life Trajectory Types and Corresponding Probabilities of Indicator Variables for People Aged 70 Years and Older: Sweden, 2018–2020**

[a]Percentages indicate means for 2018–2020.

progression" and "impaired" types, where the former had higher medical care utilization than the latter. The same distinction was made for the "dependent severe progression" and "dependent" types. In both cases, high medical care utilization was interpreted as a sign for a severe progression of 1 or more health problems.

Figure 2 depicts death counts by age and trajectory type. For women, the "terminally ill" type had the lowest median age (80.2 years), while "sudden deaths" was the type with lowest mean age among men (79.5 years). With 87.8 years for men and 91 years for women, the "dependent" type had the highest median age. Type-specific median ages were more distinct for men compared with women. Across all ages, most deaths were assigned to the "terminally ill" type for men and to the "dependent" type for women (Figure A, available as a supplement to the online version of this article at https://ajph.org), while the lowest numbers were assigned to the "sudden deaths" and "impaired" types for both women and men.

Figure 2 illustrates that trajectory types characterized by high need for elder care became more common with increasing age at death. At the highest ages, most deaths were following upon 1 of the trajectories with elder care needs. This relationship was more pronounced for women. At the modal age at death (the age when most deaths occur; age 90 years for women and 87 years for men), 5 out of 6 deaths for women and around 4 out of 5 deaths for men required elder care over the last year of life. The number of "sudden deaths" was

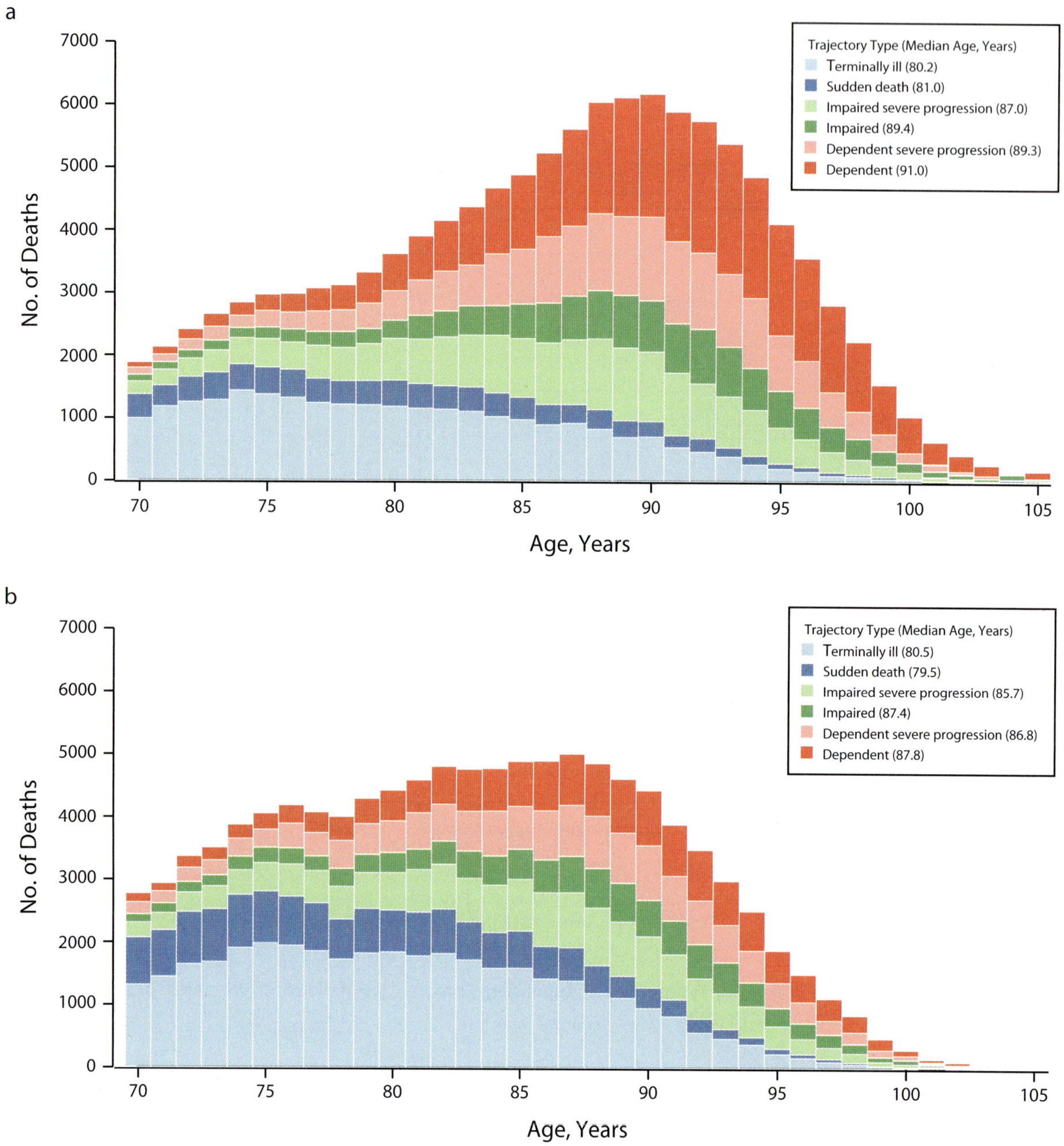

FIGURE 2— Death Counts by Age and End-of-Life Trajectory Type for People Aged 70 Years and Older by (a) Women and (b) Men: Sweden, 2018–2020

relatively stable up until age 85 years but declined thereafter and became negligible at ages 90 years and older. The "terminally ill" group reached its maximum at around age 75 and declined continuously afterward. In contrast to "sudden deaths," "terminally ill" trajectories remained at a sizable level also at ages 90 years and older.

Most deaths at younger than 80 years were assigned to trajectory types with high medical care utilization ("terminally ill," "impaired severe progression," "dependent severe progression"). For men, the share of these types remained high at ages 80 years and older, while for women, trajectories with high medical care utilization became more frequent with increasing age at death. The pattern for women was driven by the sharp increase in the number of "dependent" trajectories. For women, "dependent" and "dependent severe progression" trajectories combined constituted around half of the deaths at ages 85 to 90 years and most deaths at ages 90 years and older.

Figure 3 shows the distribution of causes of death for each trajectory type. Around half of all deaths assigned to the "terminally ill" type had a cancer as the underlying cause of death, while around half of the "sudden deaths" had a cardiovascular disease as the underlying cause of death. Both "terminally ill" and "sudden deaths" were the 2 types with the most homogenous cause-of-death profile. The "dependent" and "dependent severe progression" trajectory types had the most heterogenous cause-of-death profile, which is partially because of the high share of deaths from mental and behavioral disorders and diseases of the nervous system.

The trajectory types with high medical care utilization also had the lowest proportion of deaths from cardiovascular diseases. With a proportion between 5% and 10%, deaths from respiratory diseases encompassed a relatively constant share within each type. Deaths where the underlying cause of death was unknown were negligible in all types, but among "sudden deaths," this group included more than 5% of the deaths.

DISCUSSION

The inevitability of death is a constant that is shared by all, but the time before death looks different across persons. To the best of our knowledge, our results provide the first comprehensive analysis of the composition of end-of-life trajectories for the total population aged 70 years and older. Most existing studies on end-of-life trajectories focused on specific factors, such as number, type, or timing of care transitions,[5,6,14,18,19] or they relied on subsamples that prevented a direct link to the total population death toll.[20,21] On the basis of 2 central public health dimensions—namely elder care and medical care—we derived a data-driven classification that allowed us to illustrate the individual variation in end-of-life trajectories. Moreover, by analyzing the trajectories along gender, age, and

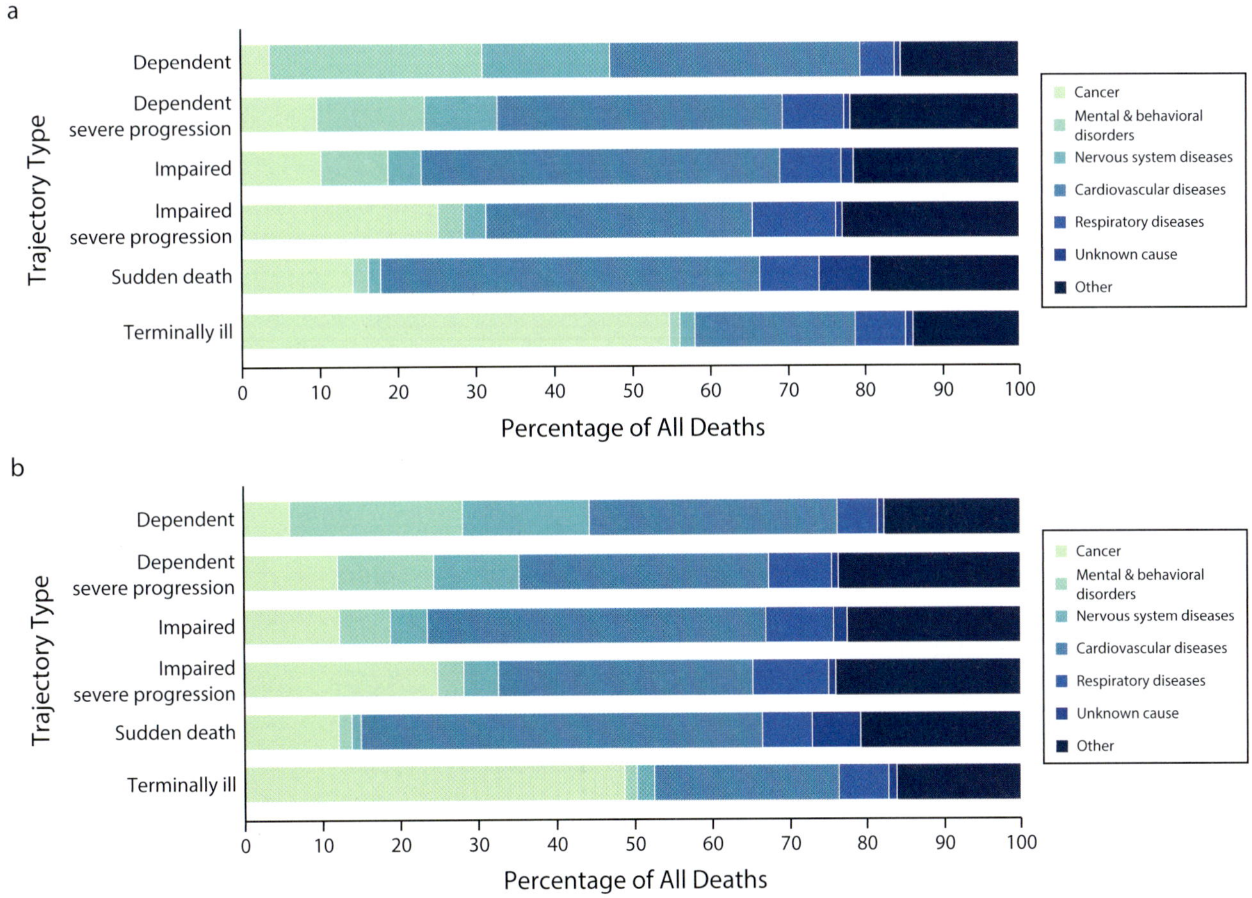

FIGURE 3— Distribution of Underlying Causes of Death by End-of-Life Trajectory Among (a) Women and (b) Men: Sweden, 2018–2020

causes of death, we gained new insights into the relationship between longevity and the end of life.

We identified 6 distinct types of end-of-life trajectories. Death counts were unevenly distributed across them. Two thirds of all deaths followed a trajectory with extensive elder care utilization throughout the last year of life, and at least half additionally showed extensive medical care utilization. The presence of extended care needs already at the beginning of the last year of life may suggest a slower progression toward death, which is different from the faster progressing "sudden death" and "terminally ill" types. Similar to Lunney et al., our classification may thus also be broadly categorized into fast and slowly progressing trajectories.[2,3]

With increasing age at death, trajectories with a comparably rapid progression toward death become less prevalent, while trajectories with a slower progression became more prevalent. The pattern may suggest that higher ages at death and, thus, longer lifespans are in part the result of a prolonged dying process. Different authors have described the prolonged dying process as a consequence of medical progress, which resulted in improved survival with diseases and, as a result, an extended period of dying by slowing the progression toward death.[22–24] Sudden unexpected deaths—previously the most common way to die[25,26]—are the smallest group in our analysis, while pathways with a slower progression are most common. This finding provides further support for the idea of a prolonged dying process. Further insights into this are required to shape the future of dying in aging societies and to meet the challenges and consequences of increasing lifespans.

End-of-life health care expenditures were and will continue to be an important aspect for health care planners because different studies concluded that the time before death comprises the highest health care costs over the life course.[8–10] Scholars also argued that a shift to long-term care becoming more frequent is likely in the future.[27] Our analysis suggests 2 important conclusions in this context. First, long-term-care settings are already the reality for most deaths in Sweden today, and, second, most deaths, particularly beyond current levels of life expectancy, follow a trajectory that could be considered relatively costly because of high elder care and medical care utilization. At this point, it is, however, not clear if an increasing number of deaths and a likely increase in lifespans will result in increasing health care expenditures in the future. The importance of future mortality improvements and probable changes in the disease panorama at the end of life have also been emphasized as pivotal factors for the future development of health care expenditures.[28,29]

The heterogeneity in cause-of-death profiles was greatest among the trajectories with the highest median age at death. Accordingly, "dependent" trajectories have the largest variation in causes of death because of a considerable share of deaths from mental and behavioral disorders and diseases of the nervous system. However, this finding must be interpreted with caution as it gets increasingly difficult to determine the cause of death at higher ages because of existing comorbidities.[30] Nevertheless, the increasing heterogeneity with age at death could indicate that end-of-life care needs vary greatly across individuals, which may be a consequence of individual disease histories becoming longer and multilayered. Findings from a Finnish study that focused on timing and place of care provision at the end of life support this hypothesis.[5]

Limitations

Despite extensive examinations that supported the plausibility of our results, our derived trajectories may be only partly generalizable to populations beyond Sweden given the variety of ways in which health care and elder care are organized. Especially medical care utilization of care home residents should be interpreted with caution as we did not have any detailed information about the care given within the care homes. In Sweden, care home residents are often only hospitalized if it is deemed unavoidable because of the high risk of unintended adverse effects, such as confusion.[31] Moreover, it is important to note that previous studies have emphasized that elder care status is a more objective measure for dependence among women compared with men because men, to a higher extent, benefit from informal caregiving of spouses.[32,33] The share of deaths following trajectories with low elder care needs could, thus, be overestimated for men.

Our analysis did not include primary care as this information is not available in nationwide registers. It will be an important future direction to also understand the role of less-severe health conditions for end-of-life trajectories. The same applies to the age range considered in this study, which was limited to deaths at ages 70 years and older. It is likely that including younger ages at death would have resulted in higher absolute and relative numbers of deaths in trajectory types with the lowest median ages at death ("terminally ill" and "sudden death"). However, given that we still included most (80%) annual deaths in Sweden, we believe that our results are based on a wide spectrum of end-of-life trajectories.

Public Health Implications

There is no consensus about the principles constituting a good death. Retaining control, being pain-free, having the choice of the place of death, and not having life prolonged pointlessly are principles that have been mentioned, among others.[34,35] Our analysis has shown that most individuals experience a last year of life with high elder care needs and medical care utilization; a pattern that becomes even more pronounced with increasing age at death. Most end-of-life trajectories that we identified may only partially align with the principles of a good death. However, as the number of deaths will rise in the future and lifespans continue to increase, it will become inevitable for societies and public health to address the question: how do we want to die? AJPH

ABOUT THE AUTHORS

Marcus Ebeling is with the Institute of Environmental Medicine, Unit of Epidemiology, Karolinska Institute, Stockholm, Sweden, and the Laboratory of Population Health, Max Planck Institute for Demographic Research, Rostock, Germany. Anna C. Meyer and Karin Modig are with the Institute of Environmental Medicine, Unit of Epidemiology, Karolinska Institute.

CORRESPONDENCE

Correspondence should be sent to Marcus Ebeling, Institute of Environmental Medicine, Unit of Epidemiology, Karolinska Institute, Box 210, 17177 Stockholm, Sweden (e-mail: marcus.ebeling@ki.se). Reprints can be ordered at https://ajph.org by clicking the "Reprints" link.

PUBLICATION INFORMATION

Full Citation: Ebeling M, Meyer AC, Modig K. Variation in end-of-life trajectories in persons aged 70 years and older, Sweden, 2018–2020. *Am J Public Health*. 2023;113(7):786–794.

Acceptance Date: March 6, 2023.

DOI: https://doi.org/10.2105/AJPH.2023.307281

CONTRIBUTORS

M. Ebeling contributed to conceptualization, formal analysis, methodology, software, validation, visualization, and writing the original draft. A. C. Meyer contributed to data curation and writing—review and editing. K. Modig contributed to conceptualization, data curation, and writing of the original draft.

ACKNOWLEDGMENTS

This work was supported by the Swedish Research Council of Health, Working Life and Welfare (FORTE; grant 2020-00028).

Earlier versions of this study have been presented at the Population Association of America Annual Meeting 2022, Atlanta, GA, and the European Population Conference 2022, Groningen, Netherlands.

Note. FORTE had no role in study design, data analysis, or preparation of the article.

CONFLICTS OF INTEREST

The authors have no relevant financial or nonfinancial interests to disclose.

HUMAN PARTICIPANT PROTECTION

This study was performed in line with the principles of the Declaration of Helsinki. The ethical approval for this study has been granted by the Regional Ethics Committee, Karolinska Institute, Stockholm, Sweden (2011/136-31/5 and 2020-04753).

REFERENCES

1. United Nations. *World Population Prospects 2019*. 2019. Available at: https://population.un.org/wpp. Accessed October 21, 2021.
2. Lunney JR, Lynn J, Foley DJ, Lipson S, Guralnik JM. Patterns of functional decline at the end of life. *JAMA*. 2003;289(18):2387–2392. https://doi.org/10.1001/jama.289.18.2387
3. Lunney JR, Lynn J, Hogan C. Profiles of older Medicare decedents. *J Am Geriatr Soc*. 2002;50(6):1108–1112. https://doi.org/10.1046/j.1532-5415.2002.50268.x
4. Raab M, Fasang A, Hess M. Pathways to death: the co-occurrence of physical and mental health in the last years of life. *Demogr Res*. 2018;38(53):1619–1634. https://doi.org/10.4054/DemRes.2018.38.53
5. Aaltonen M, Forma L, Pulkki J, Raitanen J, Rissanen P, Jylha M. Changes in older people's care profiles during the last 2 years of life, 1996–1998 and 2011–2013: a retrospective nationwide study in Finland. *BMJ Open*. 2017;7(11):e015130. https://doi.org/10.1136/bmjopen-2016-015130
6. Qureshi D, Tanuseputro P, Perez R, Seow H. Place of care trajectories in the last two weeks of life: a population-based cohort study of Ontario decedents. *J Palliat Med*. 2018;21(11):1588–1595. https://doi.org/10.1089/jpm.2018.0049
7. Meyer AC, Sandström G, Modig K. Nationwide data on home care and care home residence: presentation of the Swedish Social Service Register, its content and coverage. *Scand J Public Health*. 2022;50(7):946–958. https://doi.org/10.1177/14034948211061016
8. Howdon D, Rice N. Health care expenditures, age, proximity to death and morbidity: implications for an ageing population. *J Health Econ*. 2018;57:60–74. https://doi.org/10.1016/j.jhealeco.2017.11.001
9. Batljan I, Lagergren M. Inpatient/outpatient health care costs and remaining years of life—effect of decreasing mortality on future acute health care demand. *Soc Sci Med*. 2004;59(12):2459–2466. https://doi.org/10.1016/j.socscimed.2004.04.003
10. von Wyl V. Proximity to death and health care expenditure increase revisited: a 15-year panel analysis of elderly persons. *Health Econ Rev*. 2019;9(1):9. https://doi.org/10.1186/s13561-019-0224-z
11. Brooke HL, Talbäck M, Hörnblad J, et al. The Swedish cause of death register. *Eur J Epidemiol*. 2017;32(9):765–773. https://doi.org/10.1007/s10654-017-0316-1
12. Ludvigsson JF, Almqvist C, Bonamy AKE, et al. Registers of the Swedish total population and their use in medical research. *Eur J Epidemiol*. 2016;31(2):125–136. https://doi.org/10.1007/s10654-016-0117-y
13. Ludvigsson JF, Andersson E, Ekbom A, et al. External review and validation of the Swedish national inpatient register. *BMC Public Health*. 2011;11(1):450. https://doi.org/10.1186/1471-2458-11-450
14. Brinkman-Stoppelenburg A, Rietjens JAC, van der Heide A. The effects of advance care planning on end-of-life care: a systematic review. *Palliat Med*. 2014;28(8):1000–1025. https://doi.org/10.1177/0269216314526272
15. Teno JM, Gozalo PL, Bynum JP, et al. Change in end-of-life care for Medicare beneficiaries: site of death, place of care, and health care transitions in 2000, 2005, and 2009. *JAMA*. 2013;309(5):470–477. https://doi.org/10.1001/jama.2012.207624
16. Collins LM, Lanza ST. *Latent Class and Latent Transition Analysis: With Applications in the Social, Behavioral, and Health Sciences*. Vol 718. Hoboken, NJ: John Wiley & Sons; 2009. https://doi.org/10.1002/9780470567333
17. Weller BE, Bowen NK, Faubert SJ. Latent class analysis: a guide to best practice. *J Black Psychol*. 2020;46(4):287–311. https://doi.org/10.1177/0095798420930932
18. Aaltonen M, Rissanen P, Forma L, Raitanen J, Jylhä M. The impact of dementia on care transitions during the last two years of life. *Age Ageing*. 2012;41(1):52–57. https://doi.org/10.1093/ageing/afr133
19. Bähler C, Signorell A, Reich O. Health care utilisation and transitions between health care settings in the last 6 months of life in Switzerland. *PLoS One*. 2016;11(9):e0160932. https://doi.org/10.1371/journal.pone.0160932
20. Kaspers PJ, Pasman HRW, Onwuteaka-Philipsen BD, Deeg DJ. Changes over a decade in end-of-life care and transfers during the last 3 months of life: a repeated survey among proxies of deceased older people. *Palliat Med*. 2013;27(6):544–552. https://doi.org/10.1177/0269216312457212
21. Klinkenberg M, Visser G, Broese van Groenou MI, Van Der Wal G, Deeg DJH, Willems DL. The last

3 months of life: care, transitions and the place of death of older people. *Health Soc Care Community.* 2005;13(5):420–430. https://doi.org/10.1111/j.1365-2524.2005.00567.x

22. Rosenberg J. Whose business is dying?: Death, the home and palliative care. *Cult Stud Rev.* 2011;17(1):15–30. https://doi.org/10.5130/csr.v17i1.1971
23. Sallnow L, Smith R, Ahmedzai SH, et al. Report of the Lancet Commission on the Value of Death: bringing death back into life. *Lancet.* 2022;399(10327):837–884. https://doi.org/10.1016/S0140-6736(21)02314-X
24. Veatch RM. Choosing not to prolong dying. In: Humber JM, Almeder RF, eds. *Biomedical Ethics and the Law.* Boston, MA: Springer; 1979:517–524. https://doi.org/10.1007/978-1-4615-6561-1_34
25. Benoliel JQ, Degner LF. Institutional dying: a convergence of cultural values, technology, and social organization. In: Wass H, Neimeyer RA, eds. *Dying: Facing the Facts.* 3rd ed. New York, NY: Taylor & Francis; 1995.
26. Walter T. Historical and cultural variants on the good death. *BMJ.* 2003;327(7408):218–220. https://doi.org/10.1136/bmj.327.7408.218
27. Murphy M, Martikainen P. Use of hospital and long-term institutional care services in relation to proximity to death among older people in Finland. *Soc Sci Med.* 2013;88:39–47. https://doi.org/10.1016/j.socscimed.2013.03.042
28. Moore PV, Bennett K, Normand C. Counting the time lived, the time left or illness? Age, proximity to death, morbidity and prescribing expenditures. *Soc Sci Med.* 2017;184:1–14. https://doi.org/10.1016/j.socscimed.2017.04.038
29. Geue C, Briggs A, Lewsey J, Lorgelly P. Population ageing and healthcare expenditure projections: new evidence from a time to death approach. *Eur J Health Econ.* 2014;15(8):885–896. https://doi.org/10.1007/s10198-013-0543-7
30. Johansson LA, Björkenstam C, Westerling R. Unexplained differences between hospital and mortality data indicated mistakes in death certification: an investigation of 1,094 deaths in Sweden during 1995. *J Clin Epidemiol.* 2009;62(11):1202–1209. https://doi.org/10.1016/j.jclinepi.2009.01.010
31. Hallgren J, Ernsth Bravell M, Mölstad S, Östgren CJ, Midlöv P, Dahl Aslan AK. Factors associated with increased hospitalisation risk among nursing home residents in Sweden: a prospective study with a three-year follow-up. *Int J Older People Nurs.* 2016;11(2):130–139. https://doi.org/10.1111/opn.12107
32. Kasper JD, Pezzin LE, Rice JB. Stability and changes in living arrangements: relationship to nursing home admission and timing of placement. *J Gerontol B Psychol Sci Soc Sci.* 2010;65(6):783–791. https://doi.org/10.1093/geronb/gbq023
33. McCann M, Donnelly M, O'Reilly D. Living arrangements, relationship to people in the household and admission to care homes for older people. *Age Ageing.* 2011;40(3):358–363. https://doi.org/10.1093/ageing/afr031
34. Smith R. A good death. *BMJ.* 2000;320(7228):129–130. https://doi.org/10.1136/bmj.320.7228.129
35. Meier EA, Gallegos JV, Thomas LPM, Depp CA, Irwin SA, Jeste DV. Defining a good death (successful dying): literature review and a call for research and public dialogue. *Am J Geriatr Psychiatry.* 2016;24(4):261–271. https://doi.org/10.1016/j.jagp.2016.01.135

State Policy Removing the Personal Belief Exemption for Measles, Mumps, and Rubella (MMR) School Immunization Requirement, Washington State, 2014–2022

Tyler P. Moore, MPH, Julia C. Bennett, MSPH, Katherine Graff, BSN, RN, Mayuree Rao, MD, MS, Orvalho Augusto, MD, Helen Y. Chu, MD, MPH, Bradley H. Wagenaar, PhD, MPH, and Teal R. Bell, MPH

See also Williams and O'Leary, p. 718.

Objectives. To assess the impact of Washington State's 2019 Engrossed House Bill (EHB) 1638—which removed measles, mumps, and rubella (MMR) personal belief exemptions—on MMR vaccine series completion and exemption rates in K–12 students.

Methods. We used interrupted time-series analyses to examine changes in MMR vaccine series completion rates before and after EHB 1638 was passed and the χ^2 test for differences in exemption rates.

Results. EHB 1638 implementation was associated with a 5.4% relative increase in kindergarten MMR vaccine series completion rates (95% confidence interval = 3.8%, 7.1%; $P \le .001$), and results were similar with Oregon as a control state (no change observed in Oregon; $P = .68$). MMR exemptions overall decreased 41% (from 3.1% in 2018–2019 to 1.8% in 2019–2020; $P \le .001$), and religious exemptions increased 367% (from 0.3% to 1.4%; $P \le .001$).

Conclusions. EHB 1638 was associated with an increase in MMR vaccine series completion rates and a decrease in any MMR exemption. However, effects were partially offset by an increase in religious exemption rates.

Public Health Implications. Removal of personal belief exemptions for the MMR immunization requirement only may be an effective approach to increase MMR vaccine coverage rates statewide and among underimmunized communities. (*Am J Public Health.* 2023;113(7):795–804. https://doi.org/10.2105/AJPH.2023.307285)

AJPH July 2023, Vol 113, No. 7

State immunization laws mandating certain vaccines for school entry have been successful at achieving high immunization rates and controlling the spread of vaccine-preventable diseases.[1,2] In recent decades, however, vaccine-preventable disease outbreaks attributable to decreasing vaccination rates have occurred with increasing frequency.[3–6] In particular, measles outbreaks and continued transmission have raised concern that the United States will lose measles elimination status, which was declared in 2000.

All US states require students to be vaccinated against some diseases for school entry and allow parents to claim medical exemptions, but options for nonmedical exemptions (NMEs), such as religious or personal or philosophical beliefs (PBE), vary. Currently, 17 states allow PBEs and 44 states permit religious exemptions.[7] Although heterogeneous by state, rates of PBEs and religious exemptions have increased over the past 2 decades.[8–12] States with less restrictive exemption criteria tend to have higher rates of NMEs and lower vaccine completion rates.[9,13–15] Underimmunized populations and geographic clusters with high NME rates are at increased risk of vaccine-preventable diseases.[8,16,17]

Washington State requires that children be vaccinated against or show acquired immunity for 11 vaccine-preventable diseases before attending public or private school.[18] Until 2019, parents could waive immunization requirements by claiming 1 of 4 exemption types: medical, PBE, religious, or religious membership.[19] A religious exemption requires a parent and health care practitioner to complete and sign a certificate of exemption, and a religious membership exemption requires only a parent signature.[20,21] In Washington, NME rates increased from 3.5% in school year 2014–2015 to 4.5% in 2018–2019 primarily because of an increase in PBEs.[22] Furthermore, NME rates in Washington were substantially higher than the national median of 2.0% in school year 2017–2018.[8]

In 2019, Washington experienced 2 measles outbreaks, with the most cases (n = 87) annually in the state since 1990, highlighting the need to maintain adequate levels of population immunity to measles. The majority of cases were among unvaccinated individuals (88%), and the outbreak occurred primarily in Clark County in Southwest Washington.[17] In response, Washington legislators passed Engrossed House Bill (EHB) 1638, which aims to increase measles, mumps, and rubella (MMR) vaccine completion rates by eliminating the PBE option for the school MMR immunization requirement.[23] EHB 1638 took effect in July 2019 and required all students with a PBE for MMR to complete the vaccine series, provide evidence of acquired immunity, or claim a different exemption type at the beginning of school year 2019–2020.

Washington is the first state to remove PBEs for 1 vaccine only, and a formal evaluation of this policy is needed. The purpose of this study was to (1) assess EHB 1638's impact on MMR vaccine series completion and exemption rates, and (2) determine whether completion and exemption rate geographic patterns before passing EHB 1638 persisted following its implementation.

METHODS

We used kindergarten MMR vaccine coverage and kindergarten through 12th grade (K–12) exemption data from the Washington Annual School Immunization Report, which is managed by the Washington State Department of Health. In Washington, schools are required to report the number of students who have completed (proof of vaccination or immunity) or are exempted from (have a signed certificate of exemption) each required immunization. Additionally, schools report the number of students out of compliance (these students should be excluded from school until proof of vaccine, immunity, certificate of exemption, or initiation of an approved vaccine schedule is provided) and attending school conditionally (these students are allowed to attend school while completing required vaccines).[24] Data also include the number of students with each exemption type (i.e., medical, PBE, religious, or religious membership) and type of school (i.e., public vs private). Before school year 2019–2020, MMR vaccine completion data were collected for the kindergarten cohort and vaccine exemption data for the K–12 cohort. The Washington Annual School Immunization Report provides an annual snapshot and is primarily based on parental documentation of vaccination history.

We used annual kindergarten MMR vaccine series completion data from the Oregon School Immunization Report to use K–12 students in Oregon as a control group relative to those in Washington to assess MMR vaccine series completion rates before and after EHB 1638 implementation. We selected Oregon a priori as a control state because of its cultural and political similarity, geographic proximity to Washington, allowance of PBEs for all vaccines, and having also been affected by the 2019 measles outbreak. Oregon did not change or introduce new immunization laws during the study period.

Study Outcomes and Measures

The study period was school years 2014–2015 through 2021–2022, which includes 5 years before and 3 years after EHB 1638 implementation. Primary outcomes were kindergarten MMR vaccine series completion rates and K–12 MMR exemption rates at the state and school district levels. Secondary outcomes included K–12 exemption rates by exemption type and K–12 exemption rates and kindergarten MMR vaccine series completion rates by school type (i.e., public vs private). We included charter schools (n = 7) with public schools.

Kindergarten vaccine completion. We defined MMR vaccine series completion rate as the annual percentage of kindergarteners with documented immunity to MMR through completion of the 2-dose vaccine series or antibody titer. We used measles vaccine completion rates as a proxy for MMR vaccine completion rates after EHB 1638 implementation because of a change in data collection starting in school year 2019–2020. Separate rates for measles, mumps, and rubella were all comparable for school years 2019–2020 through 2021–2022.

K–12 vaccine exemptions. We defined MMR exemption rates as the annual percentage of K–12 students with a completed certificate of exemption for the MMR vaccine. Before the school year 2019–2020 data collection change, only the number of students with any MMR exemption (i.e., PBEs in addition to medical, religious, and religious membership exemptions) was collected. Additionally, religious, religious membership, PBE, and medical exemption data were not vaccine specific before school year 2019–2020, and we defined these exemption rates as the annual percentage of K–12 students with a completed certificate of exemption for at least 1 required vaccine for each exemption type.

Statistical Analyses

We conducted 4 interrupted time-series (ITS) analyses to estimate relative changes in kindergarten MMR vaccine completion after EHB 1638 implementation.[25] To account for overdispersion, we used negative binomial regression models and modeled the number of kindergarteners who had completed the MMR vaccination series each academic year over time with a population denominator offset (for model parameterizations, see the "Supplementary Methods" section in the Appendix, available as a supplement to the online version of this article at http://www.ajph.org).

First, we conducted an uncontrolled ITS to estimate kindergarten MMR vaccine series completion in Washington alone with a random intercept and slope for school district. We excluded school districts with less than 2 years of data from before EHB 1638 implementation or with no data from after EHB 1638 implementation (20/304 school districts). Second, we conducted a controlled ITS comparing the change in kindergarten MMR vaccine series completion rates in Washington with rates in Oregon. Third, we conducted a controlled ITS comparing the counties in Washington and Oregon directly affected by the 2019 measles outbreak: Clark County, Washington (on the Washington–Oregon border and part of the Portland, Oregon, metropolitan area), Multnomah, Washington, and Clackamas counties (Tri-County) in Oregon (the Portland, Oregon, metropolitan area). Finally, we conducted an uncontrolled ITS comparing changes in Washington kindergarten MMR vaccine series completion rates by public and private schools.

To examine changes in exemption rates following the passing of EHB 1638, we used the χ^2 test to identify significant changes in the annual rate of K–12 MMR exemptions and K–12 exemptions for any vaccine by exemption type before and after EHB 1638 implementation. We also stratified exemption rates by school type to compare differences over time between public and private schools.

To assess geographic patterns over time, we mapped school district–level kindergarten MMR vaccine series completion and K–12 exemption rates before and after EHB 1638 implementation. We used the Pearson correlation coefficient to assess the relationship between school district MMR vaccine series completion (Figure A, available as a supplement to the online version of this article at https://www.ajph.org) and exemption rates before and after EHB 1638 was passed. Additionally, we assessed the relationship between school district PBE rates before EHB 1638 implementation and the change in religious exemption rates from before to after EHB 1638 implementation. We pooled all 5 years before and all 3 years after EHB 1638 implementation for the correlation analyses. We excluded school districts that did not report data for all available years and those with errored data. We suppressed districts with fewer than 10 students from maps but included them in de-identified correlation analyses.

All reported P values are 2-sided using an $\alpha = 0.05$. We conducted analyses in SAS version 9.4 (SAS Institute, Cary, NC) and R (*R*-4.1.1, R Core Team, Vienna, Austria).

RESULTS

Before EHB 1638 passed, kindergarten MMR vaccine series completion rates were stable, without any significant annual changes ($P = .45$) and ranged between 89.5% and 90.9% from school years 2014–2015 through 2018–2019 (Table 1; Appendix Table A). After EHB 1638 implementation, kindergarten MMR vaccine series completion rates increased by 5.4% (95% confidence interval [CI] = 3.8%, 7.1%; $P \le .001$) relative to the rate before EHB 1638 implementation to 94.4% and 94.5% in school years 2019–2020 and 2020–2021, respectively, and decreased slightly to 92.6% in school year 2021–2022 ($P = .002$; Figure 1a; Table A).

Washington Versus Oregon

Results were similar when using Oregon as a control state. Washington kindergarten MMR vaccine series completion

TABLE 1— Statewide Trends in Kindergarten MMR Completion and K–12 Exemption Rates: Washington State, School Years 2014–2015 to 2021–2022

School Year	Kindergarten MMR Completion, %	K-12 Any MMR Exemption, %	K-12 Religious Exemption, %	K-12 Religious Membership Exemption, %	K-12 Medical Exemption, %	K-12 Personal Belief Exemption, %
2014–2015	89.5	3.2	0.3	0.1	1.0	3.9
2015–2016	90.9	3.0	0.3	0.1	1.0	3.8
2016–2017	90.5	3.1	0.3	0.1	1.2	3.9
2017–2018	90.7	2.9	0.3	0.1	1.0	3.7
2018–2019	90.8	3.1	0.3	0.1	0.9	3.7
2019–2020	94.4	1.8	1.4	0.2	1.0	2.9
2020–2021	94.5	1.6	1.2	0.2	0.7	2.2
2021–2022	92.7	1.7	1.4	0.2	0.7	2.0

Note. MMR = measles, mumps, and rubella. We report MMR vaccine series completion rates for kindergarteners and all exemption rates for K–12 students. Specific exemption types (i.e., religious, religious membership, medical, and personal belief) are not vaccine specific. EHB 1638 was implemented on July 28, 2019.

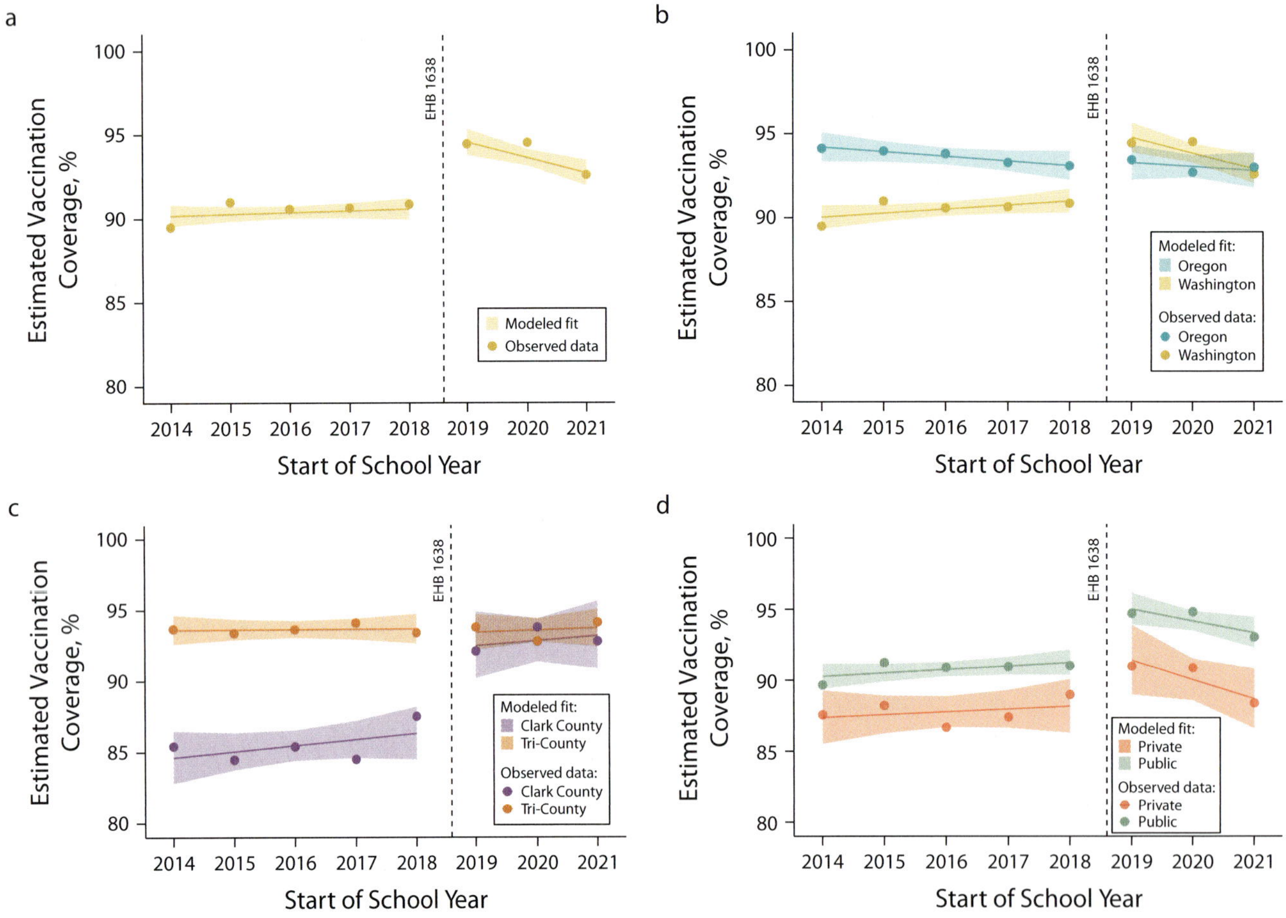

FIGURE 1— Interrupted Time-Series Estimated MMR Completion Rates Among All Kindergarten Students From School Years 2014–2015 to 2021–2022 Using Negative Binomial Regression Models for (a) Washington, (b) Washington vs Oregon, (c) Clark County, Washington, vs Tri-County, Oregon, and (d) Washington Public vs Private Schools

Note. EHB 1638 = Washington State Engrossed House Bill 1638; MMR = measles, mumps, and rubella.

rates increased 4.7% (95% CI = 1.9%, 7.6%; $P = .001$) relative to Oregon's following EHB 1638. No increase in kindergarten MMR vaccine series completion rates was observed in Oregon over the same period ($P = .68$; Figure 1b; Table A). When we restricted analyses to geographic areas affected by the 2019 measles outbreak (Clark County, Washington, and Tri-County, Oregon), kindergarten MMR vaccine series completion rates increased 7.2% (95% CI = 1.6%, 13.1%; $P = .01$) in Clark County relative to Tri-County, Oregon, and we observed no change in Tri-County, Oregon ($P = .75$; Figure 1c; Table A).

Completion in Washington by School Type

Relative changes over time in kindergarten MMR vaccine series completion rates were similar for public and private schools, although they were lower in private schools across the entire study period. Before EHB 1638 was passed, kindergarten MMR vaccine series completion rates were approximately 90% and 88% for public and private schools, respectively. Kindergarten MMR vaccine series completion rates at private schools increased by 5.3% (95% CI = 0.3%, 10.6%; $P = .04$) relative to the rate before EHB 1638, and relative increases were not significantly different between public and private schools ($P = .92$; Figure 1d; Table A).

K–12 Exemptions

Before EHB 1638 passed, annual K–12 exemption rates were relatively stable and were approximately 3.0% for any MMR exemption and approximately 0.3%, 0.1%, 1.0%, and 3.8% for religious, religious membership, medical, and personal belief exemptions, respectively, for any required vaccine (Table 1). The rate of any MMR exemption decreased by 41% relative to before EHB 1638 was passed, from 3.1% in school year 2018–2019 to 1.8% in 2019–2020 ($P \leq .001$). During the same period, the rate of students with at least 1 religious exemption for any required vaccine increased 367% relative to before EHB 1638 implementation, from 0.3% to 1.4% ($P \leq .001$), and the rate of religious membership exemptions doubled, from 0.1% to 0.2% ($P \leq .001$). By 3 years after EHB 1638 passed, religious and religious membership exemptions were stable. Overall, the rate of medical exemptions for any required vaccine did not change over the study period and was 0.9% before EHB 1638 passed in school year 2018–2019, 1.0% in 2019–2020, and 0.7% in 2020–2021 and 2021–2022.

K–12 Exemptions by School Type

Absolute decreases in any MMR exemption rates were 1.2% for both public and private schools; however, relative decreases in any MMR exemption rates were greater for public schools (41.4% relative decrease from 2.9% to 1.7%; $P \leq .001$) than for those of private schools (21.8% relative decrease from 5.5% to 4.3%; $P \leq .001$). PBE rates for any vaccine decreased to a greater degree for private (33.8% relative decrease from 6.37% to 4.22%; $P \leq .001$) than for public schools (18% relative decrease from 3.50% to 2.87%; $P \leq .001$).

Religious and religious membership exemption rates for any required vaccine increased in the year following EHB 1638 implementation for all schools but to a greater magnitude for private schools (1427% relative increase from 0.29% to 4.43%; $P \leq .001$; and 267% relative increase from 0.03% to 0.11%; $P \leq .001$, respectively) than for public schools (346% relative increase from 0.28% to 1.25% and 100% relative increase from 0.09% to 0.18%; $P \leq .001$, respectively; Appendix Table B). The rate of medical exemptions for any vaccine increased by 135.8% from 0.67% to 1.58% ($P \leq .001$) for private schools but did not meaningfully change at public schools.

School District Correlation Analyses

We included school districts that reported data for all available years (218/288) in correlation analyses. We observed geographic heterogeneity in Washington's MMR coverage and exemption rates over the entire study period. School district MMR exemption rates in school year 2018–2019 (before EHB 1638 passed) ranged from 0% to 31.2% (median = 3.3%), and in school year 2019–2020 (after EHB 1638 passed) ranged from 0% to 40.9% (median = 1.9%). MMR exemption rates before EHB 1638 implementation were positively correlated with exemption rates after EHB 1638 implementation so that school districts with higher MMR exemption rates before EHB 1638 implementation generally had higher MMR exemption rates after EHB 1638 implementation ($r = 0.83$; 95% CI = 0.79, 0.87; Figure 2a). Notably, MMR exemption rates did decrease in many school districts, with MMR exemption rates above 5% before EHB 1638 implementation, but these districts remained above the median rate after EHB 1638 implementation.

Before EHB 1638 passed, school district PBE rates for any vaccine ranged from 0% to 27.0% (median = 3.9%), and after EHB 1638 passed, they ranged from 0% to 40.0% (median = 3.3%).

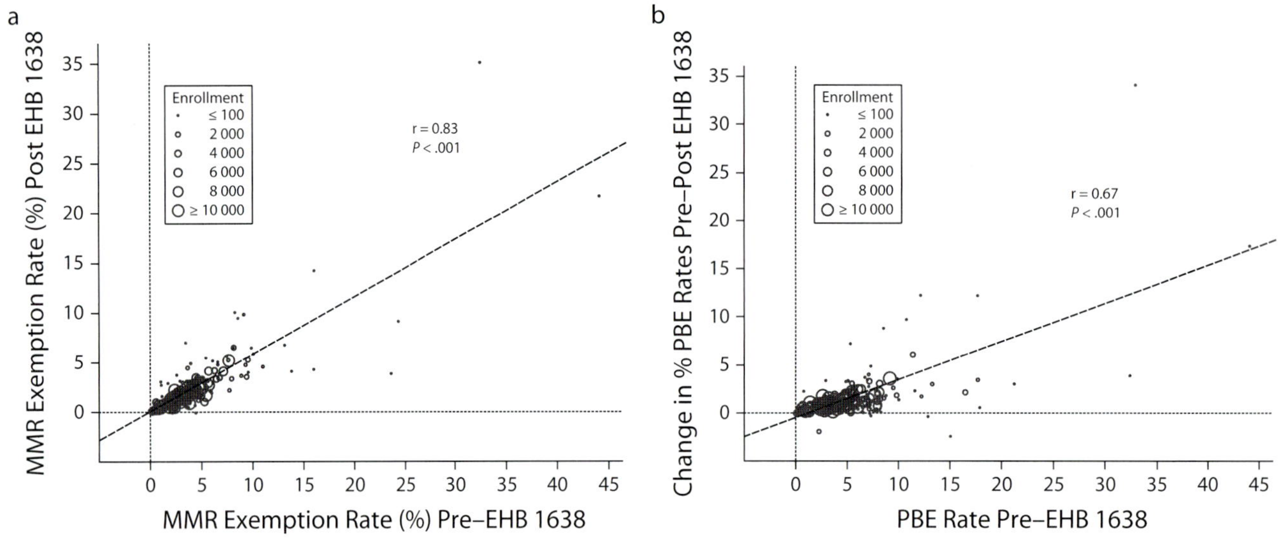

FIGURE 2— School District Correlation Analysis With Pearson Coefficient Comparing (a) K-12 Pooled MMR Exemption Rates Before and After EHB 1638 Implementation, and (b) K-12 Pooled PBE Rates Before EHB 1638 Implementation and the Change in Rate of Religious Exemptions From Before to After EHB 1638 Implementation (Pooled): School Years 2014–2015 to 2021–2022

Note. EHB 1638 = Washington State Engrossed House Bill 1638; MMR = measles, mumps, and rubella; PBE = personal belief exemption. Data points are scaled by school district enrollment in school year 2019–2020 (after EHB 1638 passed). We excluded school districts that did not report data for all available years (n = 70/288).

School district religious exemption rates for any vaccine ranged from 0% to 8.0% (median = 0.2%) before EHB 1638 implementation and 0% to 37.8% (median = 1.3%) after EHB 1638 implementation, corresponding to a 1-year relative change in school district–level religious exemption rates ranging from −3.3% to +33.2% (median change = +0.89%). School district PBE rates before EHB 1638 passed and the change in religious exemption rates from before to after EHB 1638 passed were positively correlated so that school districts with higher rates of PBEs before EHB 1638 implementation generally had larger increases in religious exemption rates (r = 0.67; CI = 0.59, 0.74; Figure 2b). Results did not change when we weighted the Pearson correlation coefficient by school district enrollment (data not shown).

In general, school district–level MMR vaccine series completion rates increased after EHB 1638 implementation, with some geographic variability. In some districts in Northeastern Washington with relatively low MMR vaccine series completion rates before EHB 1638 passed (Figure 3, panel a), MMR vaccine series completion rates increased after EHB 1638 implementation (Figure 3b), but to levels still lower than other regions of Washington. We observed similar patterns for MMR exemption rates before (Figure 3c) and after (Figure 3d) EHB 1638 implementation. Generally, higher MMR exemption rates persisted in Northeastern and Eastern Washington after EHB 1638 implementation, whereas lower MMR exemption rates were more common in Central and Western Washington after EHB 1638 implementation. We observed a somewhat similar pattern between before EHB 1638 implementation PBE rates (Figure 3e) and the change in religious exemption rates from before and after EHB 1638 implementation (Figure 3f). Higher before EHB 1638 PBE rates and greater increases in religious exemption rates from before to after EHB 1638 implementation were more common in Northeastern and Eastern Washington. However, high PBE rates before EHB 1638 implementation were also prevalent on the northern border and in Northwestern Washington, but the change in religious exemptions in these areas was mostly similar to the rest of the state.

DISCUSSION

To our knowledge, this is the first study to assess the effects of removing PBEs for only the MMR school immunization requirement. We have shown that EHB 1638 implementation was associated with a 5.4% relative increase in MMR vaccine series completion rates among kindergarteners and a decrease in the rate of any K–12 MMR exemptions in Washington State. Increases in MMR vaccine series completion rates were

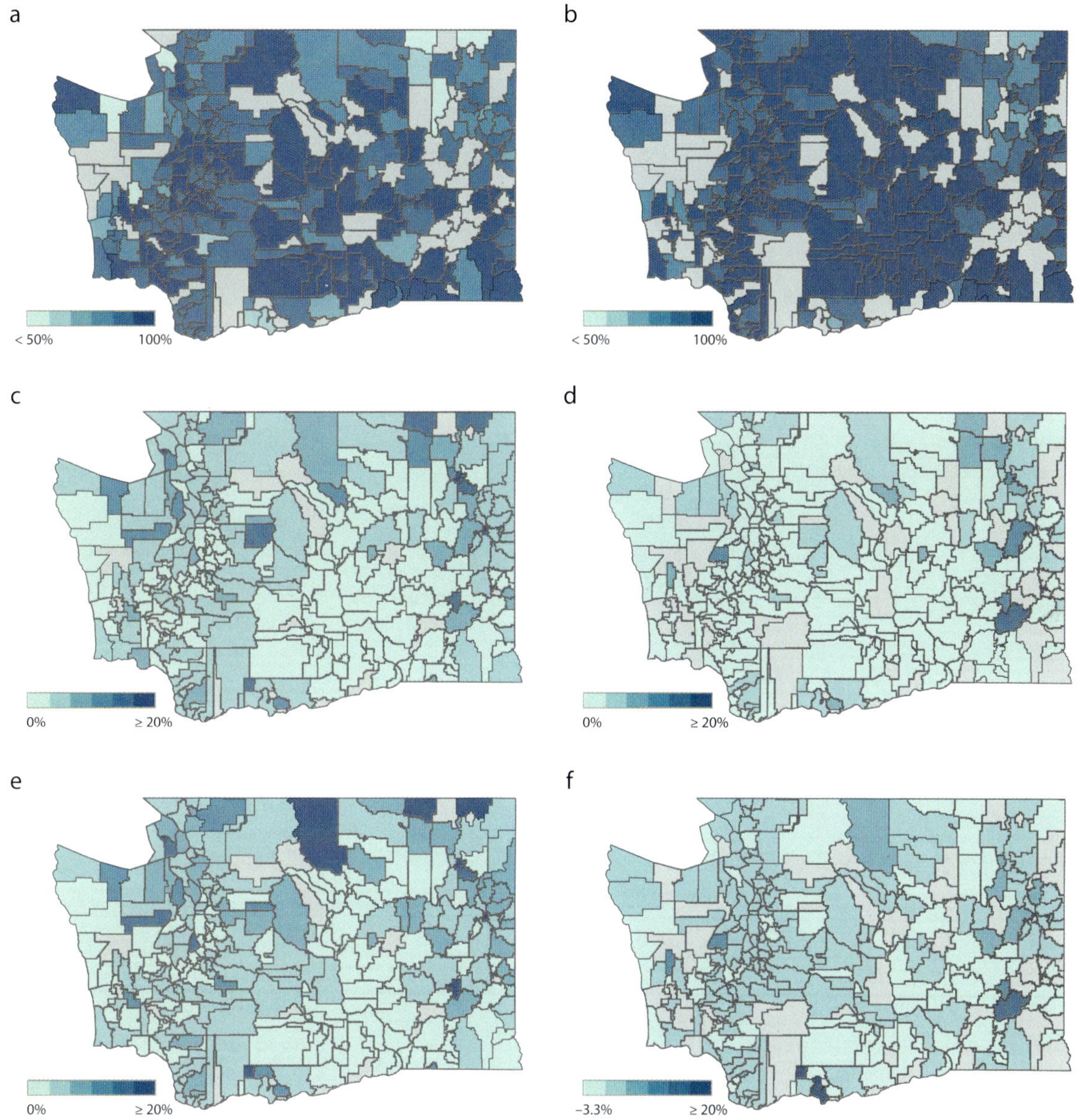

FIGURE 3— One-Year Change in MMR Completion and Exemption Rates by School District for (a) Kindergarten MMR Completion Rates Before EHB 1638 Implementation, (b) Kindergarten MMR Completion Rates After EHB 1638 Implementation, (c) K–12 MMR Exemption Rates Before EHB 1638 Implementation, (d) K–12 MMR Exemption Rates After EHB 1638 Implementation, (e) K–12 Personal Belief Exemption Rates Before EHB 1638 Implementation, and (f) Change in Religious Exemption Rates From Before and After EHB 1638 Implementation: School Years 2014–2015 to 2021–2022

Note. EHB 1638 = Washington State Engrossed House Bill 1638; MMR = measles, mumps, and rubella. Districts in gray represent those without data for the relevant year, which we excluded because of reporting errors or suppressed because student enrollment was < 10 (n = 9–64 districts excluded, depending on the year).

similar when using Oregon as a control state. Furthermore, when restricting the analysis to geographic areas in Washington and Oregon affected by the 2019 measles outbreak, MMR vaccine series completion rates increased substantially in Clark County, Washington, an area with MMR vaccine series completion rates below the state average before EHB 1638 was passed. However, MMR vaccine series completion rates did not change in Tri-County, Oregon, suggesting that the increase in MMR vaccine series completion rates observed in Washington was attributable to EHB 1638 and not in response to a perceived increase in disease risk.

Before EHB 1638 implementation, concern was raised that other exemption types may largely replace PBEs, thereby limiting the law's impact.[26]

We found that religious exemptions increased significantly, indicating that some parents sought a religious exemption in replacement of PBEs. This is despite Washington ranking toward the bottom of all US states in terms of religiosity[27] and an increasingly secular United States,[28] suggesting that religious exemptions may be held by an increasing number of individuals without such religious beliefs. These trends warrant individual-level studies to understand whether parents are seeking religious exemptions in place of the eliminated PBE options.

Unlike religious exemptions, the rate of medical exemptions did not meaningfully change statewide following EHB 1638 implementation. In addition, although the reduction in MMR exemptions was partially offset by an increase in religious exemptions, we observed a meaningful net decrease in MMR exemptions 3 years after EHB 1638 was passed. This contrasts with the situation in California, where medical exemptions and other school entry mechanisms replaced more than 70% of the decrease in NMEs after the state removed all NMEs for all vaccines.[29,30]

Given these observed replacement effects, school immunization policies must strike a balance between restricting exemption options and avoiding increases in allowed exemption types that completely offset decreases in NMEs. Our results suggest that targeted policies that allow some NMEs may be more effective than completely eliminating NMEs altogether. Other targeted policies that increase barriers to obtaining NMEs, such as required parental education, should be considered, as states with less restrictive criteria tend to have higher rates of NMEs.[13–15] Newer policies that aim to further increase the difficulty of obtaining NMEs without eliminating them altogether, such as Colorado's 2021 SB 20–163,[31] which set a 1-year expiration on NMEs, should also be evaluated to further inform optimal school immunization policies.

Importantly, we found that although private schools had lower kindergarten MMR vaccine series completion rates overall, the relative increase in MMR vaccine series completion rates after EHB 1638 implementation was significant and similar to that observed for public schools. Furthermore, MMR exemptions decreased for both public and private schools. However, religious and religious membership exemptions increased to a greater magnitude among private than among public schools, and medical exemptions increased significantly for private schools only. This aligns with findings from California, where greater increases in medical exemptions were observed for private schools.[29]

Generally, school districts with higher MMR exemption rates before EHB 1638 passed tended to have higher MMR exemption rates after EHB 1638 passed, but trends were variable. Some school districts with relatively high MMR exemption rates before EHB 1638 implementation had similarly high MMR exemption rates following EHB 1638 implementation. For many other districts, the MMR exemption rate decreased, suggesting geographic differences in EHB 1638's effect. In California, geographic regions with higher exemption rates also persisted following removal of all NMEs.[29] Additionally, school districts with higher PBE rates before EHB 1638 was passed tended to have larger increases in religious exemptions following EHB 1638 implementation, but these patterns were also variable.

Limitations and Strengths

Our study is subject to several limitations. First, because MMR exemptions by type were not collected before school year 2019–2020 and rates of specific exemption types were not vaccine specific, we were unable to assess the change in PBEs for MMR specifically. Second, although EHB 1638 implementation affected all grades, we were limited to kindergarten MMR vaccine series completion, as these data were not collected for all K–12 students before 2019. Third, only 3 years of data after EHB 1638 implementation are currently available, so we were unable to estimate long-term effects.

Last, we were not able to characterize COVID-19 pandemic impacts on student enrollment, routine health care seeking, and data collection for the Washington Annual School Immunization Report, although our use of Oregon as a control state allowed us to partially account for this external event. Nationally, COVID-19–related disruptions led to an average decrease of approximately 1% in coverage of kindergarten immunizations.[32] COVID-19 pandemic disruptions also led to delayed data collection in Washington during school years 2019–2020 and 2020–2021, the first 2 years after EHB 1638 implementation, before returning to normal reporting timelines in school year 2021–2022. This may have led to an overestimate in MMR vaccine series completion during this time. For these reasons, it is essential to continue monitoring trends in MMR vaccine series completion and exemption rates statewide and at the district level, particularly in communities with low vaccine coverage.

Nonetheless, our analysis had several strengths. Our ITS design allowed us to account for baseline trends in MMR vaccine series completion rates and use Oregon as a control state in estimating the policy's effects on MMR vaccine series completion rates. This strengthens the evidence that the increase in MMR vaccine series completion rates was attributable to EHB 1638 and not temporal trends or an increased perceived risk of measles. Furthermore, we evaluated the effects of EHB 1638 implementation on both MMR vaccine series completion rates and exemption rates by school type and school district. Our analysis has important policy and public health implications, as vaccine completion varies geographically and by school type in Washington, and geographic areas with low vaccine coverage are at the highest risk for measles outbreaks.[33,34]

Conclusions

In the first study, to our knowledge, to assess the effect of a statewide policy to remove PBEs for MMR vaccination on MMR vaccine series completion and exemption rates, we found this policy to be associated with a 5.4% relative increase in kindergarten MMR vaccine series completion rates and a 41% decrease in any MMR exemption. However, during this same period, religious exemptions significantly increased, which partially offset decreases in PBEs. Our findings suggest that eliminating PBEs while allowing other exemption types for the MMR vaccine may be an effective approach to increase MMR vaccine coverage for both public and private schools and in underimmunized communities susceptible to vaccine-preventable disease outbreaks. Continued research is needed to assess the long-term impact of this policy. AJPH

ABOUT THE AUTHORS

Tyler P. Moore, Katherine Graff, and Teal R. Bell are with the Washington State Department of Health, Tumwater. Julia C. Bennett, Mayuree Rao, Orvalho Augusto, and Bradley H. Wagenaar are with the School of Public Health, University of Washington, Seattle. Helen Y. Chu is with the Department of Medicine, University of Washington, Seattle.

CORRESPONDENCE

Correspondence should be sent to Tyler Moore, Washington State Department of Health, 111 Israel Rd SE, Tumwater, WA 98501 (e-mail: Tyler.Moore@doh.wa.gov). Reprints can be ordered at http://www.ajph.org by clicking the "Reprints" link.

PUBLICATION INFORMATION

Full Citation: Moore TP, Bennett JC, Graff K, et al. State policy removing the personal belief exemption for measles, mumps, and rubella (MMR) school immunization requirement, Washington State, 2014–2022. *Am J Public Health*. 2023;113(7): 795–804.

Acceptance Date: March 10, 2023.

DOI: https://doi.org/10.2105/AJPH.2023.307285

CONTRIBUTORS

T. P. Moore acquired the data. T. P. Moore and J. C. Bennett wrote the initial draft of the article. T. P. Moore, J. C. Bennett, K. Graff, M. Rao, O. Augusto, and T. R. Bell conceptualized and designed the study. T. P. Moore, J. C. Bennett, K. Graff, M. Rao, O. Augusto, B. H. Wagenaar, and T. R. Bell interpreted the results. T. P. Moore, J. C. Bennett, and M. Rao analyzed the data. T. P. Moore, J. C. Bennett, M. Rao, O. Augusto, H. Y. Chu, B. H. Wagenaar, and T. R. Bell revised the article.

ACKNOWLEDGMENTS

This study was funded by the Centers for Disease Control and Prevention (CDC) Immunization and Vaccines for Children Project CC3 (cooperative agreement IP19-1901).

We would like to acknowledge the Washington State Department of Health School Immunization Team for collecting and cleaning the school report data used in this analysis. Additionally, we would like to acknowledge the Oregon Health Authority, Immunization Program for providing Oregon kindergarten measles, mumps, and rubella vaccine series completion data for the controlled analyses.

Note. The content of this article is solely the responsibility of the authors and does not necessarily represent the official views of the CDC.

CONFLICTS OF INTEREST

H. Y. Chu reports consulting with Ellume, Merck, Abbvie, Pfizer, and the Bill and Melinda Gates Foundation. She has received research funding from Sanofi Pasteur and support and reagents from Ellume and Cepheid outside the submitted work. None of the other authors has any potential conflicts of interest to declare.

HUMAN PARTICIPANT PROTECTION

The Washington State institutional review board determined our evaluation of Washington State's Engrossed House Bill 1638 exempt from human participant review because no human participants were involved in this study.

REFERENCES

1. Omer SB, Salmon DA, Orenstein WA, deHart MP, Halsey N. Vaccine refusal, mandatory immunization, and the risks of vaccine-preventable diseases *N Engl J Med*. 2009;360(19):1981–1988. https://doi.org/10.1056/NEJMsa0806477
2. Orenstein WA, Hinman AR. The immunization system in the United States—the role of school immunization laws. *Vaccine*. 1999;17(suppl 3): S19–S24. https://doi.org/10.1016/S0264-410X(99)00290-X
3. Lo NC, Hotez PJ. Public health and economic consequences of vaccine hesitancy for measles in the United States. *JAMA Pediatr*. 2017;171(9): 887–892. https://doi.org/10.1001/jamapediatrics.2017.1695
4. Sundaram ME, Guterman LB, Omer SB. The true cost of measles outbreaks during the postelimination era. *JAMA*. 2019;321(12):1155–1156. https://doi.org/10.1001/jama.2019.1506
5. Salmon DA, Haber M, Gangarosa EJ, Phillips L, Smith NJ, Chen RT. Health consequences of religious and philosophical exemptions from immunization laws: individual and societal risk of measles. *JAMA*. 1999;282(1):47–53. https://doi.org/10.1001/jama.282.1.47
6. Feikin DR, Lezotte DC, Hamman RF, Salmon DA, Chen RT, Hoffman RE. Individual and community risks of measles and pertussis associated with personal exemptions to immunization. *JAMA*. 2000;284(24):3145–3150. https://doi.org/10.1001/jama.284.24.3145
7. National Conference of State Legislatures. States with religious and philosophical exemptions from school immunization requirements. 2022. Available at: https://www.ncsl.org/health/states-with-religious-and-philosophical-exemptions-from-school-immunization-requirements. Accessed April 16, 2023.
8. Bednarczyk RA, King AR, Lahijani A, Omer SB. Current landscape of nonmedical vaccination exemptions in the United States: impact of policy changes. *Expert Rev Vaccines*. 2019;18(2):175–190. https://doi.org/10.1080/14760584.2019.1562344
9. Olive JK, Hotez PJ, Damania A, Nolan MS. The state of the antivaccine movement in the United States: a focused examination of nonmedical exemptions in states and counties. *PLoS Med*. 2018;15(6):e1002578. [Erratum in: *PLoS Med*. 2018;15(7):e1002616]. https://doi.org/10.1371/journal.pmed.1002578
10. Delamater PL, Leslie TF, Yang YT. Examining the spatiotemporal evolution of vaccine refusal: nonmedical exemptions from vaccination in California, 2000–2013. *BMC Public Health*. 2018;18(1):458. https://doi.org/10.1186/s12889-018-5368-y

11. Richards JL, Wagenaar BH, Van Otterloo J, et al. Nonmedical exemptions to immunization requirements in California: a 16-year longitudinal analysis of trends and associated community factors. *Vaccine.* 2013;31(29):3009–3013. https://doi.org/10.1016/j.vaccine.2013.04.053
12. Williams JTB, Rice J, Cox-Martin M, Bayliss EA, O'Leary ST. Religious vaccine exemptions in kindergartners: 2011–2018. *Pediatrics.* 2019;144(6):e20192710. https://doi.org/10.1542/peds.2019-2710
13. Omer SB, Pan WK, Halsey NA, et al. Nonmedical exemptions to school immunization requirements: secular trends and association of state policies with pertussis incidence. *JAMA.* 2006;296(14):1757–1763. https://doi.org/10.1001/jama.296.14.1757
14. Shaw J, Mader EM, Bennett BE, Vernyi-Kellogg OK, Yang YT, Morley CP. Immunization mandates, vaccination coverage, and exemption rates in the United States. *Open Forum Infect Dis.* 2018;5(6):ofy130. https://doi.org/10.1093/ofid/ofy130
15. Blank NR, Caplan AL, Constable C. Exempting schoolchildren from immunizations: states with few barriers had highest rates of nonmedical exemptions. *Health Aff (Millwood).* 2013;32(7):1282–1290. https://doi.org/10.1377/hlthaff.2013.0239
16. Omer SB, Enger KS, Moulton LH, Halsey NA, Stokley S, Salmon DA. Geographic clustering of nonmedical exemptions to school immunization requirements and associations with geographic clustering of pertussis. *Am J Epidemiol.* 2008;168(12):1389–1396. https://doi.org/10.1093/aje/kwn263
17. Washington State Department of Health. Measles in Washington, 2019. *epiTrends.* 2019;24(9). Available at: https://doh.wa.gov/sites/default/files/legacy/Documents/5000//420-002-epitrends2019-09.pdf. Accessed May 19, 2022.
18. Washington State Legislature. Vaccine-preventable diseases children must be protected against for full immunization. 2014. Available at: https://apps.leg.wa.gov/wac/default.aspx?cite=246-105-030. Accessed April 16, 2023.
19. Washington State Legislature. Immunization program—exemptions. 2019. Available at: https://apps.leg.wa.gov/rcw/default.aspx?cite=28A.210.090. Accessed April 16, 2023.
20. Washington State Department of Health. School and childcare immunization. Available at: https://doh.wa.gov/community-and-environment/schools/immunization#:~:text=Washington%20State%20Law%20allows%20parents,exempted%20for%20personal%2Fphilosophical%20reasons. Accessed July 12, 2022.
21. Washington State Legislature. Required documentation of immunization status. 2019. Available at: https://app.leg.wa.gov/wac/default.aspx?cite=246-105-050. Accessed April 16, 2023.
22. Centers for Disease Control and Prevention. Vaccination coverage and exemptions among kindergartners. May 14, 2021. Available at: https://www.cdc.gov/vaccines/imz-managers/coverage/schoolvaxview/data-reports/index.html?CDC_AA_refVal=https%3A%2F%2Fwww.cdc.gov%2Fvaccines%2Fimz-managers%2Fcoverage%2Fschoolvaxview%2Fdata-reports%2Fexemptions-reports%2F2016-17.html. Accessed April 16, 2023.
23. Washington State Legislature. HB 1638—2019-20. Promoting immunity against vaccine preventable diseases. 2019. Available at: https://app.leg.wa.gov/billsummary?BillNumber=1638&Year=2019. Accessed April 16, 2023.
24. Washington State Legislature. Duties of schools and childcare centers. 2019. Available at: https://app.leg.wa.gov/wac/default.aspx?cite=246-105-060. Accessed April 20, 2023.
25. Xiao H, Augusto O, Wagenaar BH. Reflection on modern methods: a common error in the segmented regression parameterization of interrupted time-series analyses. *Int J Epidemiol.* 2020;50(3):1011–1015. https://doi.org/10.1093/ije/dyaa148
26. Delamater PL, Omer SB. Legislative and administrative actions to increase vaccination coverage in Washington schools. *Hum Vaccin Immunother.* 2020;16(5):1171–1177. https://doi.org/10.1080/21645515.2019.1678358
27. Lipka M, Wormald B. How religious is your state? 2016. Available at: https://www.pewresearch.org/fact-tank/2016/02/29/how-religious-is-your-state/?state=Washington. Accessed April 16, 2023.
28. Pew Research Center. Modeling the future of religion in America. 2022. Available at: https://www.pewresearch.org/religion/2022/09/13/modeling-the-future-of-religion-in-america. Accessed April 16, 2023.
29. Delamater PL, Pingali SC, Buttenheim AM, Salmon DA, Klein NP, Omer SB. Elimination of nonmedical immunization exemptions in California and school-entry vaccine status. *Pediatrics.* 2019;143(6):e20183301. https://doi.org/10.1542/peds.2018-3301
30. Nyathi S, Karpel HC, Sainani KL, et al. The 2016 California policy to eliminate nonmedical vaccine exemptions and changes in vaccine coverage: an empirical policy analysis. *PLoS Med.* 2019;16(12):e1002994. https://doi.org/10.1371/journal.pmed.1002994
31. SB 20-163—School entry immunization. Colorado General Assembly. 2020. Available at: https://leg.colorado.gov/bills/sb20-163. Accessed April 16, 2023.
32. Centers for Disease Control and Prevention. Vaccination coverage with selected vaccines and exemption rates among children in kindergarten—United States, 2020–21 school year. *MMWR Morb Mortal Wkly Rep.* 2022;71(16):561–568. https://doi.org/10.15585/mmwr.mm7116a1
33. Lieu TA, Ray GT, Klein NP, Chung C, Kulldorff M. Geographic clusters in underimmunization and vaccine refusal. *Pediatrics.* 2015;135(2):280–289. https://doi.org/10.1542/peds.2014-2715
34. Wolf E, Rowhani-Rahbar A, Tasslimi A, Matheson J, DeBolt C. Parental country of birth and childhood vaccination uptake in Washington State. *Pediatrics.* 2016;138(1):e20154544. https://doi.org/10.1542/peds.2015-4544

Using Modernized Medicaid Data to Advance Evidence-Based Improvements in Maternal Health

Jamie R. Daw, PhD, Samantha G. Auty, MS, Lindsay K. Admon, MD, MSc, and Sarah H. Gordon, PhD

Medicaid is the primary payor for nearly half of all births in the United States and plays a disproportionate role in covering maternity care for low-income people, rural people, and minoritized racial groups.

Newly available, modernized Medicaid claims data—the Transformed Medicaid Statistical Information System Analytic Files (TAF)—offer a significant opportunity to conduct novel research that can drive the development of evidence-based programs and policies for Medicaid beneficiaries before, during, and after pregnancy. Yet, the public health research community has so far underused the TAF for maternal health research.

We provide an overview of the TAF and how they compare to other major data sets available to study maternal health. We highlight some major limitations of the TAF and offer strategies to maximize the potential of these novel data to accelerate timely, rigorous research to improve maternal health and health equity. (*Am J Public Health*. 2023;113(7):805–810. https://doi.org/10.2105/AJPH.2023.307287)

AJPH July 2023, Vol 113, No. 7

The United States has the highest maternal mortality rate among comparable countries.[1] Furthermore, structural racism and systemic barriers to high-quality health care have contributed to longstanding racial and socioeconomic disparities in maternal health.[1] Medicaid pays for nearly half of US births and plays a disproportionate role in covering maternity care for low-income people, rural people, and minoritized racial groups.[2] Thus, addressing adverse pregnancy outcomes in Medicaid is fundamental to reducing maternal health inequities.

State Medicaid programs are acting as laboratories for change, approaching this challenge in unique ways. Examples of state initiatives include pregnancy-related Medicaid extensions to 12 months postpartum, coverage for doula care, increased reimbursement for nurse midwives, and alternative maternity care payment models.[2] Key stakeholders, including Medicaid agencies, maternal mortality review committees, and perinatal quality collaboratives, have emphasized the urgent need for timely, high-quality data to build the evidence base for maternal health innovations and policies.[3] Additionally, the National Institutes of Health recently announced an agency-wide maternal health initiative,[4] and several foundations are prioritizing actionable maternal health research.[5]

In 2019, the Centers for Medicare & Medicaid Services (CMS) released new data that respond to these calls: the Transformed Medicaid Statistical Information System Analytic Files (TAF). The TAF are a major modernization of Medicaid claims and offer a new opportunity for research to improve services for pregnant and postpartum Medicaid beneficiaries. Yet, the TAF have so far been underused by the maternal health research community, potentially because of lack of awareness, cost, data storage and management, or methodological concerns. We provide an overview of the TAF and how they compare to other major national data sets to study maternal health. We also outline practical strategies to overcome the data's limitations.

OVERVIEW

From 1999 to 2015, CMS compiled state Medicaid claims submissions into the Medicaid Analytic eXtract (MAX). Although MAX data have been used in many previous studies on important maternal health issues, their potential was limited by data quality, state inconsistencies, and long lags in data availability.[6] Researchers have also used raw Medicaid data obtained directly from individual states with varying quality and usability and limited ability to conduct cross-state comparisons. In 2019, CMS released the TAF—the next generation of research-ready Medicaid data—the result of a lengthy effort to improve the standardization and quality of Medicaid claims.[6,7] The TAF contain demographic, eligibility, and enrollment information, as well as 4 claims files that include encounters financed by fee-for-service and managed care: (1) inpatient care, (2) long-term care and mental health facilities, (3) prescription drugs and durable medical equipment, and (4) other services (i.e., physician services, outpatient care, some inpatient claims, dental, and labs).

Compared with the retired MAX files, the TAF have automated uniform processing across states, resulting in a significant improvement in quality and usability, particularly for research focused on national estimates or state-level comparisons. The TAF are also timelier (submitted monthly vs quarterly), provide more information on encounters in managed care (which covered 72% of Medicaid beneficiaries in 2020[8]), and include more than 1000 additional data elements (e.g., "other" fee-for-service claims, capitated payments, managed care encounters, supplemental payments). Moreover, TAF beneficiary IDs allow tracking beneficiaries over time and across states and linkage to other federal data. TAF data quality is also more transparent; CMS contracts with Mathematica to maintain the Data Quality Atlas, an online dashboard that evaluates the quality of TAF data elements by state and year through comparison with external benchmarks.[9]

As of February 2023, the TAF are available for all Medicaid beneficiaries in all 50 states, the District of Columbia, and Puerto Rico from 2016 to 2020.[7] TAF data application forms are available on the CMS Research Data Assistance Center Web site.[7] CMS estimates a 20-week timeline from application to data delivery. There are 2 options for data access: (1) purchase a seat through the CMS Virtual Research Data Center for an annual fee of $15 000 to $22 000, or (2) purchase physical TAF data for a fee based on the number of files and cohort size requested.[10] Reusing a physical extract for a new project costs $2000 and is free for those writing doctoral dissertations. Purchasing physical files can cost less and allows more flexible institutional use and reuse but requires researchers to maintain their own secure data infrastructure.

OTHER DATA SOURCES COMPARED

Table 1 provides a brief overview of the major national data sources for US maternal health research. We do not review electronic health records, given their lack of national scope, nor commercial claims, given their underrepresentation of publicly insured populations most affected by maternal health inequities. By complementing the gaps in existing data sources, the TAF have the potential to spark new avenues for maternal health research, particularly on the causes and consequences of maternal health inequities and the impact of state-level Medicaid policies. Importantly, the TAF contain longitudinal data on health care from all settings (not only inpatient or at childbirth), thus expanding the type and timing of maternal health exposures and outcomes that can be studied on a large scale. These advantages are balanced by several key limitations, which we will describe, that are critical for maternal health researchers to consider and address.

IDENTIFYING BIRTHS

Using the TAF for maternal health research requires accurate identification of pregnancy-related events. There are established algorithms for identifying live births in inpatient claims data using diagnosis and procedure codes, including by CMS specifically for the TAF.[11–15] However, in our own work with the TAF, we encountered 2 key issues in applying these algorithms. First, birth claims can be found in the inpatient file only, the other services file only, or both. In the TAF 2016 through 2018, we found that 12% of birth claims were only in the other services file. Existing algorithms are designed for inpatient claims and thus may inaccurately identify births in the other services file. Thus, researchers should exclude any codes unrelated to live birth or delivery (e.g., those specific to the postpartum period) for application to the other services file. The most recently published CMS technical specifications for identifying live births also exclude these codes, reflecting this concern.[14,15]

Second, although published algorithms (including CMS' most recent) often include newborn *International Classification of Diseases, 10th Revision* (Geneva, Switzerland: World Health Organization; 1992 [*ICD-10*]) codes (e.g., Z38), many states use the same beneficiary ID for a mother and a child younger than 1 year. To prevent misidentification of newborn claims as maternal claims and inaccurate assessment of birth timing, use of newborn

TABLE 1— Multistate and National Data Sources for Maternal Health Research: United States, February 2023

Data Source (Steward)	Data Type	Population (Sample)	Advantages	Disadvantages
PRAMS (CDC)	Survey	Representative multistate sample (46 states in 2020, n ≈ 50 000 births annually)	Representative sample Includes some birth certificate variables Includes all patients regardless of payer Contains demographics, social determinants, health care utilization, and some health outcomes Contains state identifiers No cost	State participation varies over time Sample sizes limit subgroup analyses Limited follow-up period and focus on prenatal period Limited health outcomes Self-reported outcomes Excludes nonlive births
Natality Files (CDC)	Administrative (birth certificates)	99% of US live births (n ≈ 4 million births annually)	Population based Includes all patients regardless of payer Contains demographic and clinical birth outcomes at delivery Publicly available at the state level No cost	Limited to delivery outcomes Limited maternal health outcomes No diagnosis or procedure codes Excludes nonlive births County-level data require lengthy access process
SID/NIS (HCUP)	Administrative (inpatient discharges)	SID is 97% of US community hospital discharges (NIS is 20% sample of SID)	Large representative sample Includes all patients regardless of payer Contains diagnosis and procedure codes to measure inpatient health care utilization and outcomes SID contains state identifiers	Limited to inpatient encounters (delivery and readmission) Limited demographics and poor capture of race/ethnicity High cost
TAF (CMS)	Administrative (claims)	100% of Medicaid claims (n ≈ 1.5 million births annually)	Population based Contains diagnosis and procedure codes to measure health care utilization and outcomes for all health care types and settings Includes maternity and nonmaternity care before, during, and after pregnancy, allowing for longitudinal study Contains state and zip code identifiers, allowing comparisons across states and links to area-level variables Links to other federal surveys and administrative data	Quality of demographic data can be low and varies across states Some data harmonization issues across states Bundled payment codes can mask receipt of individual perinatal services Beneficiary disenrollment can create challenges for longitudinal studies Delivery-related services in "other" services create challenges for applying established inpatient algorithms for identifying births and birth outcomes No family identifier to study maternal–infant dyad Moderate to high cost

Note. CDC = Centers for Disease Control and Prevention; CMS = Centers for Medicare & Medicaid Services; HCUP = Healthcare Cost and Utilization Project; NIS = National Inpatient Sample; PRAMS = Pregnancy Risk Assessment Monitoring System; SID = state inpatient databases; TAF = Transformed Medicaid Statistical Information System Analytic Files.

codes should be carefully considered when identifying deliveries in the TAF—particularly for state-years with moderate to high levels of shared maternal–infant IDs (34 states in 2016).[16]

Researchers can validate their chosen approach for identifying live births in the TAF using Centers for Disease Control and Prevention (CDC) Natality data, which capture 99% of US live births. Using the publicly available CDC Wide-Ranging Online Data for Epidemiologic Research (WONDER) online tool, researchers can generate state-year– or state-month–level counts of live births when Medicaid was the primary payer. These gold standard counts can then be compared with live birth counts based on algorithms applied to the TAF. For example, in our work with the 2016 to 2018 TAF, we found that inclusion of newborn codes resulted in a significant overcount of Medicaid-paid live births relative to expected counts from the CDC WONDER.

CMS has also published algorithms for identifying miscarriage, stillbirth, and termination in the TAF.[15] Although validation is more difficult for TAF users to conduct themselves, given the lack of population-based external benchmarks for these outcomes, other studies have found high validity of claims-based measures for identifying nonlive births compared with medical records.[17] As for any claims data, the TAF cannot be used to identify pregnancy events with no health care contact (e.g., home births, many early pregnancy losses).

MEASURING OUTCOMES AND UTILIZATION

The TAF contain dates of service, diagnostic codes, and procedure codes to measure maternal health conditions, health care utilization, and health outcomes. Diagnostic codes from delivery claims can be used to estimate week of gestation with high validity when compared with obstetric estimates[18] and thus can be used to construct periods corresponding to pregnancy, preconception, and postpartum, during which care and outcomes can be longitudinally measured.

The potential to use the TAF to track patients over time comes with an important limitation. For studies that require long periods of enrollment (e.g., 1 year or more preconception or postpartum), researchers will have to restrict study cohorts to continuously enrolled beneficiaries. This may affect generalizability, particularly in Medicaid nonexpansion states (i.e., where fewer low-income adults qualify for Medicaid outside pregnancy), for people with incomes near the eligibility thresholds, and for immigrants who may qualify for maternity care under Medicaid state rules but not otherwise. Despite this limitation, as we will outline, the TAF present a unique opportunity to study long-term outcomes and sequalae after pregnancy, and, conversely, to explore how preconception health care and health affect pregnancy outcomes.

Health Conditions and Outcomes

TAF data can be used to measure health risks among pregnant Medicaid beneficiaries and identify high-risk groups. Existing algorithms for identifying chronic conditions, pregnancy complications, and clinical risk factors can be applied to the TAF based on claims from preconception, pregnancy, delivery, and postpartum. To measure infant and maternal mortality, the TAF's enrollment file includes date of death for all beneficiaries. The TAF can also be linked to the National Death Index segment (accessible through a virtual research data center), which includes the underlying conditions and *ICD-10* and CDC category codes for cause of death. Other claims-based maternal health outcomes can be measured in the TAF, including severe maternal morbidity (SMM), interpregnancy intervals, and postpartum mood and anxiety disorders.

Researchers should ensure that algorithms to identify outcomes are applied appropriately given the unique structure of the TAF; for example, guidelines published by the CDC and CMS to measure SMM recommend using data in both the inpatient and other services files but include codes designed for delivery-related inpatient claims. Measures of SMM may need to be modified to accurately detect SMM in the TAF's other services file.[13,19] For example, SMM *ICD-10* codes for sepsis include T81.4 "infection following a procedure," which may not indicate a morbid event in the outpatient setting (e.g., wound infection or mastitis), resulting in overcounts of SMM. Similarly, in states with maternal–infant ID sharing, SMM indicators such as ventilation could indicate a newborn service, resulting again in overcounts of SMM. There is an urgent need for development and validation of additional claims-based measures for maternal health outcomes beyond SMM, particularly those that may present in the outpatient setting.

Health Care Utilization

The TAF contain detailed health services utilization for inpatient care, long-term care, outpatient care, and prescription drugs. Although the CDC Natality files have long included measures of prenatal care (month of first visit, total number of visits), recent research has shown how claims data can measure perinatal health care receipt, content, timing, and quality in far more detail.[20,21]

One significant caveat to the potential of the TAF (or any claims data) to measure perinatal services is the increased use of bundled maternity payments (typically covering delivery and routine prenatal and postpartum care). Bundled payment procedure codes are typically issued at the time of delivery, and thus individual perinatal services may not be accurately reflected in claims. Therefore, CMS advises that TAF users exclude deliveries with a bundled payment code.[22] Alternatively, users can limit the states included in their analysis to address this issue (14 states had < 5% of deliveries with bundled payment in 2020).[9]

However, bundled payments present an issue only for research focused on measuring routine services included in the bundle. Indeed, the TAF could be very useful for conducting evaluations of alternative payment models, even if some perinatal services cannot be disaggregated. For example, researchers could compare changes in cesarean delivery rates (which have a unique bundled payment code) or outcomes in periods not covered by the bundle (e.g., health care utilization and outcomes in the postpartum year) in states that implemented alternative payments compared with those that did not. Despite CMS' blanket guidance, exclusion of births or states with bundled payment codes in the TAF should be based on the research question of interest.

Relatedly, one advantage of the TAF is that they allow maternal health research to extend beyond routine prenatal and postpartum care, including connections to primary and specialty care before, after, and between pregnancies. Health care utilization and quality measures can further be connected to long-term patient outcomes, which has previously not been possible with Natality or inpatient discharge data. Building a comprehensive picture of health care patterns for Medicaid beneficiaries and the implications for maternal health and disparities would be invaluable for informing state Medicaid programs, public health planning, and clinical practice.

MEASURING MATERNAL HEALTH INEQUITIES

The TAF contain only a limited set of variables for measuring maternal health inequities, including race and ethnicity, age, language, citizenship, disability indicators, income, zip code, and veteran status.[23] Maternal health researchers should be aware that the quality of race/ethnicity data in the TAF is low for the majority of states. However, CMS is actively working on improvements, so researchers must assess data quality on a state-year basis. Researchers studying live births can evaluate the quality of the TAF race/ethnicity data by comparing state-year– or state-month–level Medicaid-paid live birth counts by race/ethnicity in the CDC WONDER to live birth counts by race/ethnicity in the TAF. Researchers should set an a priori threshold for state-year inclusion based on concordance of these counts (e.g., 20% absolute difference). For studies of other pregnancy events and for sociodemographic variables not contained in the CDC WONDER, researchers should use the Data Quality Atlas to assess data quality, which generally compares state-year–level TAF estimates for each demographic element to external benchmarks from the American Community Survey.

The National Center of Health Statistics data linkage program offers a promising avenue for researchers to overcome the current limitations of TAF data quality. This program allows individual-level linkage of the TAF to other federal survey and administrative data, which could facilitate novel research on disparities, social determinants, and a wide range of health and social outcomes not captured in claims.[24] The National Health Interview Survey, the National Health and Nutrition Examination Survey, and the National Hospital Care Survey have been successfully linked to the TAF, and more linkages will be developed. With these linkages and approximately 1.5 million births annually, the TAF have a large enough sample size to apply intersectionality frameworks that interrogate how multiple overlapping social identities correlate with pregnancy outcomes. Researchers can also use state, county, and zip codes to directly link the TAF to area-level variables that capture upstream determinants of health, such as area-level measures of structural racism,[25] providing additional insight into the systemic mechanisms underlying maternal health inequities.[25]

STUDYING THE MATERNAL–INFANT DYAD

The current structure of the TAF presents challenges for studying the maternal–infant dyad. In states with maternal–infant ID sharing, claims for the mother and infant cannot be differentiated except for services that are always provided to mothers only (e.g., Z30—contraception counseling) or newborns only (e.g., Z00.11—newborn health examination). For states without ID sharing, there is currently no mechanism to link maternal and infant claims in the TAF. Although many states assign a unique family identifier to related beneficiaries, CMS does not currently provide this in the TAF. This should be a priority for future TAF improvements.

CONCLUSIONS

Despite limitations, modernized Medicaid claims data provide an important opportunity to inform evidence-based programs and policies to improve maternal health and health equity. Ongoing data improvements and methodological research are urgently needed to accelerate the use of these new data, including validated claims-based cohort and outcome definitions. With these tools in hand, the public health community will be in a better position to contribute evidence to address one of the United States' most significant and intractable public health problems. AJPH

ABOUT THE AUTHORS

Jamie R. Daw is with the Department of Health Policy and Management, Columbia University Mailman School of Public Health, New York, NY. Samantha G. Auty and Sarah H. Gordon are with the Department of Health Law, Policy and Management, Boston University School of Public Health, Boston, MA. Lindsay K. Admon is with the Department of Obstetrics and Gynecology and the Institute for Healthcare Policy and Innovation, University of Michigan, Ann Arbor.

CORRESPONDENCE

Correspondence should be sent to Jamie R. Daw, 722 W 168th St, New York, NY 10032 (e-mail: jrd2199@columbia.edu). Reprints can be ordered at http://www.ajph.org by clicking the "Reprints" link.

PUBLICATION INFORMATION

Full Citation: Daw JR, Auty SG, Admon LK, Gordon SH. Using modernized Medicaid data to advance evidence-based improvements in maternal health. *Am J Public Health*. 2023;113(7):805–810.

Acceptance Date: March 13, 2023.

DOI: https://doi.org/10.2105/AJPH.2023.307287

CONTRIBUTORS

J. R. Daw conceptualized the study and completed the initial draft. J. R. Daw, L. K. Admon, and S. H. Gordon acquired funding. S. G. Auty, L. K. Admon, and S. H. Gordon contributed to writing, editing, and revising. All authors approved the final version of the article.

ACKNOWLEDGMENTS

This work was primarily supported by the Commonwealth Fund Medicaid Grant Program (grant 20213011). S. G. Auty was separately supported by the Agency for Healthcare Research and Quality and the National Center for Advancing Translational Sciences.

S. H. Gordon is a senior advisor in the US Department of Health and Human Services.

Note. The findings and views in this article do not reflect the official views or policy of the US Department of Health and Human Services.

CONFLICTS OF INTEREST

The authors have no conflicts of interest to declare.

HUMAN PARTICIPANT PROTECTION

This article is not human participant research, so institutional review board approval was not required.

REFERENCES

1. DeClerque E, Zephyrin L. Maternal mortality in the United States: a primer. 2020. Available at: https://doi.org/10.26099/ta1q-mw24. Accessed March 27, 2023.
2. Medicaid and CHIP Payment and Access Commission. Medicaid's role in maternal health. 2020. Available at: https://www.macpac.gov/publication/chapter-5-medicaids-role-in-maternal-health. Accessed January 18, 2022.
3. Chappel A, DeLew N, Grigorescu V, Smith SR. Addressing the maternal health crisis through improved data infrastructure: guiding principles for progress. *Health Affairs Forefront*. 2021. Available at: https://doi.org/10.1377/forefront.20210729.265068. Accessed March 27, 2023.
4. National Institutes of Health. Implementing a Maternal Health and Pregnancy Outcomes Vision for Everyone (IMPROVE) initiative. Available at: https://www.nih.gov/research-training/medical-research-initiatives/improve-initiative. Accessed March 18, 2022.
5. Prina L. Maternal health: what funders have been supporting. *Health Aff (Millwood)*. 2021;40(4):675–676. https://doi.org/10.1377/hlthaff.2021.00350
6. Shapiro WL. Catalyzing the future of Medicaid research: the T-MSIS analytic files. 2022. Available at: https://www.ashecon.org/newsletter/catalyzing-the-future-of-medicaid-research-the-t-msis-analytic-files. Accessed September 6, 2022.
7. Centers for Medicare & Medicaid Services. Transformed Medicaid Statistical Information System (T-MSIS) Analytic Files (TAF). 2022. Available at: https://www.medicaid.gov/medicaid/data-systems/macbis/medicaid-chip-research-files/transformed-medicaid-statistical-information-system-t-msis-analytic-files-taf/index.html. Accessed February 7, 2023.
8. Kaiser Family Foundation. Total Medicaid MCO enrollment. August 4, 2022. Available at: https://www.kff.org/other/state-indicator/total-medicaid-mco-enrollment. Accessed February 7, 2023.
9. Centers for Medicare & Medicaid Services. Data Quality Atlas. 2022. Available at: https://www.medicaid.gov/dq-atlas/welcome. Accessed September 6, 2022.
10. Research Data Assistance Center. CMS fee information for CMS research identifiable data. 2023. Available at: https://resdac.org/cms-fee-information-research-identifiable-data. Accessed February 7, 2023.
11. Clapp MA, James KE, Friedman AM. Identification of delivery encounters using *International Classification of Diseases, Tenth Revision*, diagnosis and procedure codes. *Obstet Gynecol*. 2020;136(4):765–767. https://doi.org/10.1097/AOG.0000000000004099
12. Heins SE, Faherty LJ, Kranz AM. A comparison of approaches to identify live births using the Medicaid analytic extract. *Health Serv Outcomes Res Methodol*. 2022;22(1):49–58. https://doi.org/10.1007/s10742-021-00252-w
13. Centers for Medicare & Medicaid Services. Identifying beneficiaries with severe maternal morbidity (SMM): technical specifications. 2021. Available at: https://www.medicaid.gov/medicaid/data-and-systems/downloads/macbis/smm_techspecs.docx. Accessed March 27, 2023.
14. Centers for Medicare & Medicaid Services. Maternal and infant health (MIH): identifying pregnant and postpartum beneficiaries: reference codes. 2021. Available at: https://www.medicaid.gov/medicaid/data-and-systems/downloads/macbis/mih_reference_codes.xlsx. Accessed March 27, 2023.
15. Centers for Medicare & Medicaid Services. Maternal and infant health (MIH): identifying pregnant and postpartum beneficiaries in administrative data: technical specifications. 2021. Available at: https://www.medicaid.gov/medicaid/data-and-systems/downloads/macbis/mih_techspecs.docx. Accessed March 27, 2023.
16. Centers for Medicare & Medicaid Services. Use of the same Medicaid identification number for mother and newborn services in 2016. 2021. Available at: https://www.medicaid.gov/dq-atlas/downloads/supplemental/7011_Shared_Medicaid_IDs_2016.pdf. Accessed March 27, 2023.
17. Zhu Y, Bateman BT, Hernandez-Diaz S, et al. Validation of claims-based algorithms to identify non-live birth outcomes. *Pharmacoepidemiol Drug Saf*. 2023;32(4):468–474. https://doi.org/10.1002/pds.5574
18. Leonard SA, Panelli DM, Gould JB, Gemmill A, Main EK. Validation of *ICD-10-CM* diagnosis codes for gestational age at birth. *Epidemiology*. 2023;34(1):64–68. https://doi.org/10.1097/EDE.0000000000001557
19. Centers for Disease Control and Prevention. How does CDC identify severe maternal morbidity? 2019. Available at: https://www.cdc.gov/reproductivehealth/maternalinfanthealth/smm/severe-morbidity-ICD.htm. Accessed February 8, 2023.
20. Gourevitch RA, Natwick T, Chaisson CE, Weiseth A, Shah NT. Variation in guideline-based prenatal care in a commercially insured population. *Am J Obstet Gynecol*. 2022;226(3):413.e1–413.e19. https://doi.org/10.1016/j.ajog.2021.09.038
21. Steenland M, Kozhimannil K, Werner E, Daw J. Health Care use by commercially insured postpartum and nonpostpartum women in the United States. *Obstet Gynecol*. 2021;137(5):782–790. https://doi.org/10.1097/AOG.0000000000004359
22. Centers for Medicare & Medicaid Services. Bundled payment for prenatal care. 2022. Available at: https://www.medicaid.gov/dq-atlas/downloads/data_by_topic/TAF_dataquality_Bundled_Pmts_Prenatal/TAF_dataquality_Bundled_Pmts_Prenatal.pdf. Accessed October 4, 2022.
23. Saunders H, Chidambaram P. Medicaid administrative data: challenges with race, ethnicity, and other demographic variables. April 28, 2022. Available at: https://www.kff.org/medicaid/issue-brief/medicaid-administrative-data-challenges-with-race-ethnicity-and-other-demographic-variables. Accessed September 12, 2022.
24. Centers for Disease Control and Prevention. NCHS data linkage activities. 2022. Available at: https://www.cdc.gov/nchs/data-linkage/index.htm. Accessed November 1, 2022.
25. Hardeman RR, Homan PA, Chantarat T, Davis BA, Brown TH. Improving the measurement of structural racism to achieve antiracist health policy. *Health Aff (Millwood)*. 2022;41(2):179–186. https://doi.org/10.1377/hlthaff.2021.01489

Examining Smoking Prevalence Disparities in Virginia Counties by Rurality, Appalachian Status, and Social Vulnerability, 2011–2019

Asal Pilehvari, PhD, Wen You, PhD, Rebecca A. Krukowski, PhD, and Melissa A. Little, PhD, MPH

Objectives. To estimate county-level cigarette smoking prevalence in Virginia and examine cigarette use disparities by rurality, Appalachian status, and county-level social vulnerability.

Methods. We used 2011–2019 Virginia Behavioral Risk Factor Surveillance System proprietary data with geographical information to estimate county-level cigarette smoking prevalence using small area estimation. We used the Centers for Disease Control and Prevention's social vulnerability index to quantify social vulnerability. We used the 2-sample statistical *t* test to determine the differences in cigarette smoking prevalence and social vulnerability between counties by rurality and Appalachian status.

Results. The absolute difference in smoking prevalence was 6.16 percentage points higher in rural versus urban counties and 7.52 percentage points higher in Appalachian versus non-Appalachian counties in Virginia ($P < .001$). Adjusting for county characteristics, a higher social vulnerability index is associated with increased cigarette use. Rural Appalachian counties had 7.41% higher cigarette use rates than did urban non-Appalachian areas. Tobacco agriculture and a shortage of health care providers were significantly associated with higher cigarette use prevalence.

Conclusions. Rural Appalachia and socially vulnerable counties in Virginia have alarmingly high rates of cigarette use. Implementation of targeted intervention strategies could reduce cigarette use, ultimately reducing tobacco-related health disparities. (*Am J Public Health*. 2023;113(7):811–814. https://doi.org/10.2105/AJPH.2023.307298)

AJPH July 2023, Vol 113, No. 7

Cigarette smoking remains the leading cause of preventable morbidity and mortality in the United States.[1] Although the prevalence of current cigarette smoking among US adults has decreased over the past several decades to 13.7% in 2018,[2] this decrease has not been as pronounced in rural areas,[3] such as rural Appalachia (as high as 33% in some counties).[4] The Appalachian region, which extends across 13 states, has historically been characterized by its mountainous terrain, poverty, limited health care access, and reliance on tobacco agriculture and coal mining, which may contribute to elevated smoking rates. Smokers living in rural Appalachia are more likely to smoke earlier in life and to smoke more heavily, and they are less likely to successfully quit.[3,4] Consequently, smokers in Appalachia are disproportionately affected by smoking-related illnesses.[5]

Although individual (e.g., attitudes, beliefs) and socioeconomic (e.g., education, income, occupation) factors have been used to explain smoking patterns across the United States,[6] much less is known about environmental factors. The Centers for Disease Control and Prevention developed the social vulnerability index (SVI), which evaluates 4 spheres of influence on health: (1) socioeconomic status, (2) household composition and disability, (3) minority status and language, and (4) housing type and transportation. These components are closely tied to a population's health care access and adherence to health guidelines, which may affect the effectiveness of tobacco control initiatives in rural areas with scarce resources or areas with a high SVI. Although the SVI has been studied extensively with natural disasters and disease outbreaks, we are not aware of any studies that have investigated the association between SVI and cigarette use and how it differs by rurality and Appalachian status.

Disentangling predictors and drivers of tobacco use disparities is a vital step toward promoting tobacco-related health equity. We aimed to fill this gap by examining and comparing county-level disparities in cigarette smoking prevalence by rurality, Appalachian status, and SVI score in Virginia. Specifically, we hypothesized that rural counties, Appalachian counties, and counties with higher SVI scores would have higher cigarette use prevalence. Furthermore, we hypothesized that rural Appalachian counties with a higher SVI score would have the highest prevalence rate.

METHODS

We estimated county-level cigarette smoking prevalence using Virginia Behavioral Risk Factor Surveillance System (BRFSS) data, which surveyed approximately 8832 respondents, representing the approximately 7 million Virginian adults, annually between 2011 and 2019. BRFSS is designed to produce reliable estimates at the state level; however, sample sizes for counties are too small to provide representative area-level estimates. Therefore, to estimate smoking prevalence rates at the county level, we used the small area estimation method.[7] To obtain reliable estimates for counties with missing or small sample sizes, we followed standard procedure and combined BRFSS data from 2011 to 2019 into 3 periods of 3 years each (2011–2013, 2014–2016, 2017–2019). We incorporated survey weights into all analyses.

We defined smokers as adults who reported having smoked more than 100 cigarettes in their lifetime and a current smoking frequency of "every day" or "some days." We classified counties using the 2013 rural–urban continuum codes, with code values 1 to 3 classified as urban and code values 4 to 9 classified as rural.[8] We determined whether a county was Appalachian or non-Appalachian based on the Appalachian Regional Commission database.[9]

We used the SVI to identify counties' social vulnerability levels[10] through 15 social factors across 4 dimensions of vulnerability (range = 0–1, with higher values indicating more vulnerability). We compared current smoking prevalence between rural versus urban and between Appalachian versus non-Appalachian counties using the 2-sample *t* test. We analyzed the impact of SVI level and the combination of rurality with Appalachian status on county-level cigarette smoking prevalence, controlling for factors such as coal mining, tobacco agriculture, and health care provider shortages using multivariate regression analysis with robust SEs. We mapped SVI with estimated current smoking prevalence along with rural identifiers on Virginia counties using Census shape data files. We performed analyses and mapping in Stata version 16 (StataCorp LP, College Station, TX).

RESULTS

Virginia comprises 133 counties, including 80 (60.15%) urban and 53 (39.85%) rural counties, of which 25 (18.8%) are in the Appalachian region (including 17 rural Appalachian and 8 urban Appalachian). Average SVI level in Virginia was 0.49, whereas average SVI level in rural areas was 0.63 compared with 0.40 in urban areas ($P < .001$). We found no statistically significant difference in SVI score between Appalachian and non-Appalachian counties (0.51 vs 0.50). However, average SVI score in rural Appalachian counties was higher than in urban Appalachian counties (0.58 vs 0.35; $P < .001$).

Overall cigarette smoking prevalence in Virginia was 14.80%, whereas cigarette use prevalence among rural counties was 19.38% compared with 13.20% in urban counties (difference = 6.16 percentage points; $P < .001$). Moreover, cigarette use was significantly higher in Appalachian (20.89%) compared with non-Appalachian (13.37%) counties (difference = 7.52 percentage points; $P < .001$). Overall, the highest cigarette smoking prevalence was seen in rural Appalachian counties (mean = 22.47%). There were 28 counties in Virginia with a cigarette smoking prevalence higher than 20% and an average SVI score of 0.62 (located in the third quartile of SVI distribution). Of these, the majority were classified as rural (71.43% rural and 35.80% rural Appalachian).

Figure 1 demonstrates the association of high SVI level with high cigarette smoking rates in counties across Virginia for the period of 2017 to 2019. Adjusting for county characteristics, a higher SVI level is associated with increased cigarette use. Rural Appalachian counties had 7.41 percentage points higher cigarette use rates than did urban non-Appalachian areas. Tobacco agriculture and a shortage of health care providers were also significantly associated with higher SVI level

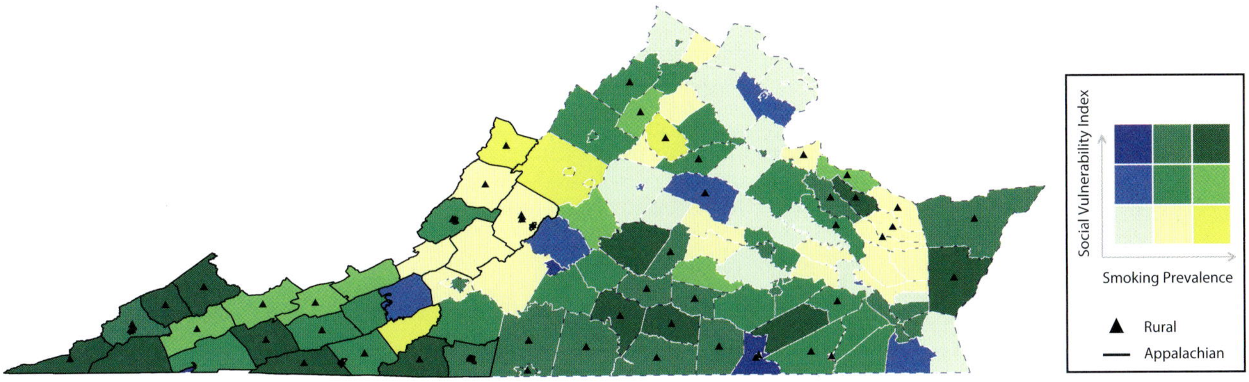

FIGURE 1— Association of Smoking Prevalence and Social Vulnerability by Rurality and Appalachian Status: Virginia Counties, 2017–2019

Note. We estimated current cigarette smoking prevalence using the small area estimation method. The US Centers for Disease Control and Prevention developed the social vulnerability index; a higher social vulnerability index refers to higher vulnerability. We based urban–rural classifications on the 2013 urban–rural continuum codes developed by the Department of Agriculture and the Rural Health Research Center.[8] Counties with code values of 1–3 are classified as urban, and those with code values of 4–9 are considered as rural. We obtained county centroid locations from US Census Bureau shapefiles.

and being an Appalachian county (Tables A and B, available as a supplement to the online version of this article at http://www.ajph.org).

DISCUSSION

Current cigarette smoking rates in Virginia were close to the national average[11]; however, rates are much higher in rural counties, especially in rural Appalachian counties, signaling the heightened need for action in those areas. Furthermore, rural counties had the highest SVI scores, which also corresponded with higher smoking prevalence. Despite rural Appalachian counties having the highest cigarette smoking rates in Virginia, they did not have the highest SVI levels. We found that tobacco agriculture and lack of health care providers were significantly associated with cigarette smoking prevalence. Further research is needed to examine whether other factors, such as pro-tobacco culture, or multidimensional indexes, such as social deprivation index, also play roles in the high cigarette use rates in rural Appalachia.

Furthermore, it is also possible that the SVI level does not adequately capture the unique social vulnerability characteristics of rural Appalachia. For instance, despite it having a high level of poverty, 84% of the population is non-Hispanic White, and multiunit housing is not common in this region.[12] Because these factors make up 2 dimensions of the SVI, the association of SVI score with smoking prevalence by rurality and Appalachian status in our study warrants further investigation to identify the role each dimension of the SVI plays in the elevated smoking prevalence in rural Appalachia. Our findings further underscore the need for both smoking prevention and cessation programs in the rural Appalachian counties of Virginia.

PUBLIC HEALTH IMPLICATIONS

Although smoking has been decreasing over the past decade, residents in rural Appalachian counties of Virginia exhibit alarmingly high rates of cigarette smoking, which likely will result in remarkable and yet preventable health and economic consequences. Implementation of targeted, evidence-based interventions is warranted to reduce tobacco-related disease faced by rural Appalachian residents. Strategies should provide incentives to farmers to grow economically sustainable alternatives to tobacco, increase access to cessation resources in counties with health care shortages, and target campaigns for rural communities on the dangers of tobacco.[5] AJPH

ABOUT THE AUTHORS

All authors are with the Department of Public Health Science, University of Virginia, and University of Virginia Comprehensive Cancer Center, Charlottesville.

CORRESPONDENCE

Correspondence should be sent to Asal Pilehvari, Technical Director of Population Health and Cancer Outcomes Core, Department of Public Health Science, University of Virginia Comprehensive Cancer Center, 560 Ray C Hunt Dr, Room 2107, Charlottesville, VA 22908 (e-mail: asal@virginia.edu). Reprints can be ordered at http://www.ajph.org by clicking the "Reprints" link.

PUBLICATION INFORMATION

Full Citation: Pilehvari A, You W, Krukowski RA, Little MA. Examining smoking prevalence disparities in Virginia counties by rurality, Appalachian status, and social vulnerability, 2011–2019. *Am J Public Health*. 2023;113(7):811–814.

Acceptance Date: March 19, 2023.

DOI: https://doi.org/10.2105/AJPH.2023.307298

CONTRIBUTORS

A. Pilehvari and W. You performed the data analyses. All authors contributed to the study design and initial and final drafts of the article.

ACKNOWLEDGMENTS

This work was supported by the Cancer Control and Population Health program at the University of Virginia Cancer Center, provided through the National Institutes of Health Cancer Center Support (grant P30CA044579) and the National Cancer Institute (award R01CA267963). The Population Health and Cancer Outcomes Core at the University of Virginia Comprehensive Cancer Center provided percent effort funding support and access to proprietary Behavioral Risk Factor Surveillance System data.

Note. The content of this article is solely the responsibility of the authors and does not necessarily represent the official views of these funding agencies.

CONFLICTS OF INTEREST

The authors have no conflicts of interest to disclose.

HUMAN PARTICIPANT PROTECTION

No protocol approval was necessary because no human participants were involved in this study.

REFERENCES

1. US Department of Health and Human Services. *The Health Consequences of Smoking—50 Years of Progress: A Report of the Surgeon General.* Atlanta, GA: Centers for Disease Control and Prevention; 2014.
2. Centers for Disease Control and Prevention. Tobacco product use and cessation indicators among adults—United States, 2018. *MMWR Morb Mortal Wkly Rep.* 2019;68(45):1013–1019. https://doi.org/10.15585/mmwr.mm6845a2
3. Ziller EC, Lenardson JD, Paluso NC, Talbot JA, Daley A. Rural–urban differences in the decline of adolescent cigarette smoking. *Am J Public Health.* 2019;109(5):771–773. https://doi.org/10.2105/AJPH.2019.304995
4. Cardarelli K, Westneat S, Dunfee M, May B, Schoenberg N, Browning S. Persistent disparities in smoking among rural Appalachians: evidence from the Mountain Air Project. *BMC Public Health.* 2021;21(1):1–12. https://doi.org/10.1186/s12889-021-10334-6
5. Beatty K, Hale N, Meit M; Appalachian Regional Commission. Health disparities related to smoking in Appalachia, practical strategies and recommendations for communities. April 2019. Available at: https://www.arc.gov/wp-content/uploads/2020/06/HealthDispairitiesRelatedtoSmokinginAppalachiaApr2019.pdf. Accessed April 6, 2023.
6. US Department of Health and Human Services. *Smoking Cessation: A Report of the Surgeon General.* 2020. Available at: https://www.hhs.gov/sites/default/files/2020-cessation-sgr-full-report.pdf. Accessed April 6, 2023.
7. Rao JNK, Molina I. *Small Area Estimation.* Hoboken, NJ: Wiley; 2015. https://doi.org/10.1002/9781118735855
8. US Department of Agriculture, Economics Research Services. The 2013 urban–rural continuum codes. 2020. Available at: https://www.ers.usda.gov/data-products/rural-urban-continuum-codes.aspx. Accessed April 6, 2023.
9. Appalachian Regional Commission. Appalachian counties. 2022. Available at: https://www.arc.gov/appalachian-counties-served-by-arc. Accessed April 6, 2023.
10. Centers for Disease Control and Prevention, Agency for Toxic Substances and Disease Registry. CDC/ATSDR social vulnerability index. November 16, 2022. Available at: https://www.atsdr.cdc.gov/placeandhealth/svi/index.html. Accessed April 6, 2023.
11. Centers for Disease Control and Prevention. Current cigarette use among adults (Behavior Risk Factor Surveillance System) 2018. March 17, 2022. Available at: https://www.cdc.gov/tobacco/data_statistics/fact_sheets/adult_data/cig_smoking/index.htm. Accessed April 6, 2023.
12. Pollard K, Jacobsen LA. The Appalachian Region: a data overview from the 2016–2020 American Community Survey. September 27, 2022. Available at: https://www.arc.gov/report/the-appalachian-region-a-data-overview-from-the-2016-2020-american-community-survey. Accessed April 6, 2023.

Evaluation of Public Health Contact Tracing for Mpox Among Gay, Bisexual, and Other Men Who Have Sex With Men—10 US Jurisdictions, May 17–July 31, 2022

Anna Barry Cope, PhD, Robert D. Kirkcaldy, MD, Paul J. Weidle, PharmD, David A. Jackson, MD, Nicholas Laramee, MPH, Robyn Weber, MPH, Julia Rowse, MPH, Anil Mangla, PhD, Brian Fox, MA, MPH, Katharine E. Saunders, DNP, Kristen Taniguchi, Lauren Usagawa, Megan E. Cahill, PhD, Pauline Harrington, MPH, Erin K. Ricketts, MD, Khalil Harbi, MSPH, Lenka Malec, MPH, Tingting Gu Templin, PhD, Dan Drociuk, Terri Hannibal, MSN, Rachel Klos, DVM, and Kyle T. Bernstein, PhD

See also Pitts et al., p. 729.

Objectives. To examine the potential impact of contact tracing to identify contacts and prevent mpox transmission among gay, bisexual, and other men who have sex with men (MSM) as the outbreak expanded.

Methods. We assessed contact tracing outcomes from 10 US jurisdictions before and after access to the mpox vaccine was expanded from postexposure prophylaxis for persons with known exposure to include persons at high risk for acquisition (May 17–June 30, 2022, and July 1–31, 2022, respectively).

Results. Overall, 1986 mpox cases were reported in MSM from included jurisdictions (240 before expanded vaccine access; 1746 after expanded vaccine access). Most MSM with mpox were interviewed (95.0% before vaccine expansion and 97.0% after vaccine expansion); the proportion who named at least 1 contact decreased during the 2 time periods (74.6% to 38.9%).

Conclusions. During the period when mpox cases among MSM increased and vaccine access expanded, contact tracing became less efficient at identifying exposed contacts.

Public Health Implications. Contact tracing was more effective at identifying persons exposed to mpox in MSM sexual and social networks when case numbers were low, and it could be used to facilitate vaccine access. (*Am J Public Health*. 2023;113(7):815–818. https://doi.org/10.2105/AJPH.2023.307301)

AJPH July 2023, Vol 113, No. 7

Contact tracing is used to interrupt transmission of infectious diseases, including mpox, by identifying exposed persons (contacts) so that they can receive prevention services. The success of contact tracing in preventing transmission largely depends on how many patients' contacts are identified and reported during interviews with health department staff.

During the 2022 US outbreak, the first case of mpox was confirmed on May 17, 2022.[1] Daily case counts peaked at 631 on August 1, 2022.[2] Most mpox cases occurred among gay, bisexual, and other men who have sex with men (MSM) and were attributed to sexual or close intimate contact during the 3 weeks before symptom onset.[3] JYNNEOS vaccine supply was initially limited, and health departments prioritized access for postexposure prophylaxis for persons aged 18 years or older named as contacts by persons with mpox. On June 28, 2022, access was expanded to include persons aged 18 years or older at high risk for acquiring mpox.[4] We sought to examine the potential impact of contact tracing among MSM to identify contacts and prevent mpox transmission in 10 US jurisdictions before and after vaccine access expanded.

METHODS

Ten US jurisdictions (Colorado, District of Columbia, Florida, Hawaii, Idaho, Michigan, New York City, North Carolina, South Carolina, Wisconsin) provided aggregated contact tracing data for mpox cases among MSM aged 18 years or older diagnosed during May 17 through July 31, 2022. Jurisdictions provided the numbers of MSM with mpox who were reported, were interviewed, named at least 1 contact with whom they had close physical contact within 21 days after symptom onset, and named at least 1 sexual contact with whom they engaged in sex or other intimate contact within 21 days after symptom onset. Total numbers of named contacts, named sexual contacts, and unnamed contacts (insufficient information was available to initiate follow-up) were also provided.

We stratified data by the period before (May 17–June 30, 2022) and after (July 1–31, 2022) access to the JYNNEOS vaccine was expanded.[4] We calculated contact indices (the number of contacts divided by the number of interviewed MSM with mpox) for all named contacts, named sexual contacts, and unnamed contacts.

RESULTS

In participating jurisdictions, 240 (12%) mpox cases among MSM were reported before vaccine access expansion and 1746 (88%) were reported after vaccine access expansion. Case investigators interviewed similar proportions of persons during both periods (95.0% and 97.0%, respectively; Figure 1).

Case investigators elicited locating information for at least 1 named contact from 179 (74.6%) patients before vaccine access expansion and 679 (38.9%) afterward. Similarly, case investigators elicited at least 1 named sexual contact from 92 (38.3%) patients before vaccine access expansion and 473 (27.1%) after expansion.

Case investigators obtained locating information for 754 named contacts before vaccine access expansion (107 [14%] were sexual contacts) and 1378 named contacts after access expansion, including 317 (23%) sexual contacts. The named contact index decreased from 3.31 before vaccine access expansion (when case counts were low) to 0.81 after expansion. The named sexual contact index was less than 1 during both periods and decreased from 0.47 before vaccine access expansion to 0.19 after expansion. MSM with mpox reported 341 (42.1%) unnamed contacts during interviews before vaccine access expansion and 469 (57.9%) afterward. The unnamed contact index decreased from 1.50 before vaccine access expansion to 0.28 afterward.

DISCUSSION

Although health department staff interviewed most mpox patients among MSM, identifying their contacts became more challenging as the number of mpox cases and investigator workload increased and vaccine access expanded beyond named contacts. In this analysis, more than half of MSM with mpox did not provide locating information for any contacts. Without such information, health departments cannot notify contacts of exposure, limiting the ability to reduce transmission. Additional public health strategies beyond contact tracing, such as vaccination and behavior change recommendations,[5] might be needed to reduce mpox transmission among MSM.

Contact tracing for other sexually transmitted diseases often has low reporting rates of sexual partners.[6–10] An estimated 80% of the partners of syphilis patients are either unreported or not found because health departments lack sufficient locating information.[6] In our evaluation, we did not assess reasons why mpox patients did not name contacts. For sexually transmitted diseases (and as might be the case with mpox), patients may be unable to name sexual partners because encounters were anonymous or facilitated by dating Web sites and apps.[8,9] Patients may prefer to notify partners themselves, desire privacy, or believe there is little value in participating in public health–sponsored contact tracing.[9,10]

Several jurisdictions anecdotally described patients providing locating information for persons from their social and sexual networks to facilitate access to the vaccine even after access was expanded. However, the observed reduction in the reporting of named contacts after expanded vaccine availability suggests this practice was infrequent. The proportion of MSM patients naming contacts might have been artificially inflated early in the outbreak to facilitate vaccine access, contributing to an apparent decrease in naming contacts once vaccine access expanded. Reductions in the proportion of MSM with mpox who named a nonsexual or sexual contact after vaccine expansion resulted in fewer than 1 named contact per interviewed mpox patient. During periods of increased transmission, contact indices less than 1 suggest that contact tracing alone will be insufficient to reduce incidence within a community.

The Centers for Disease Control and Prevention developed messaging for

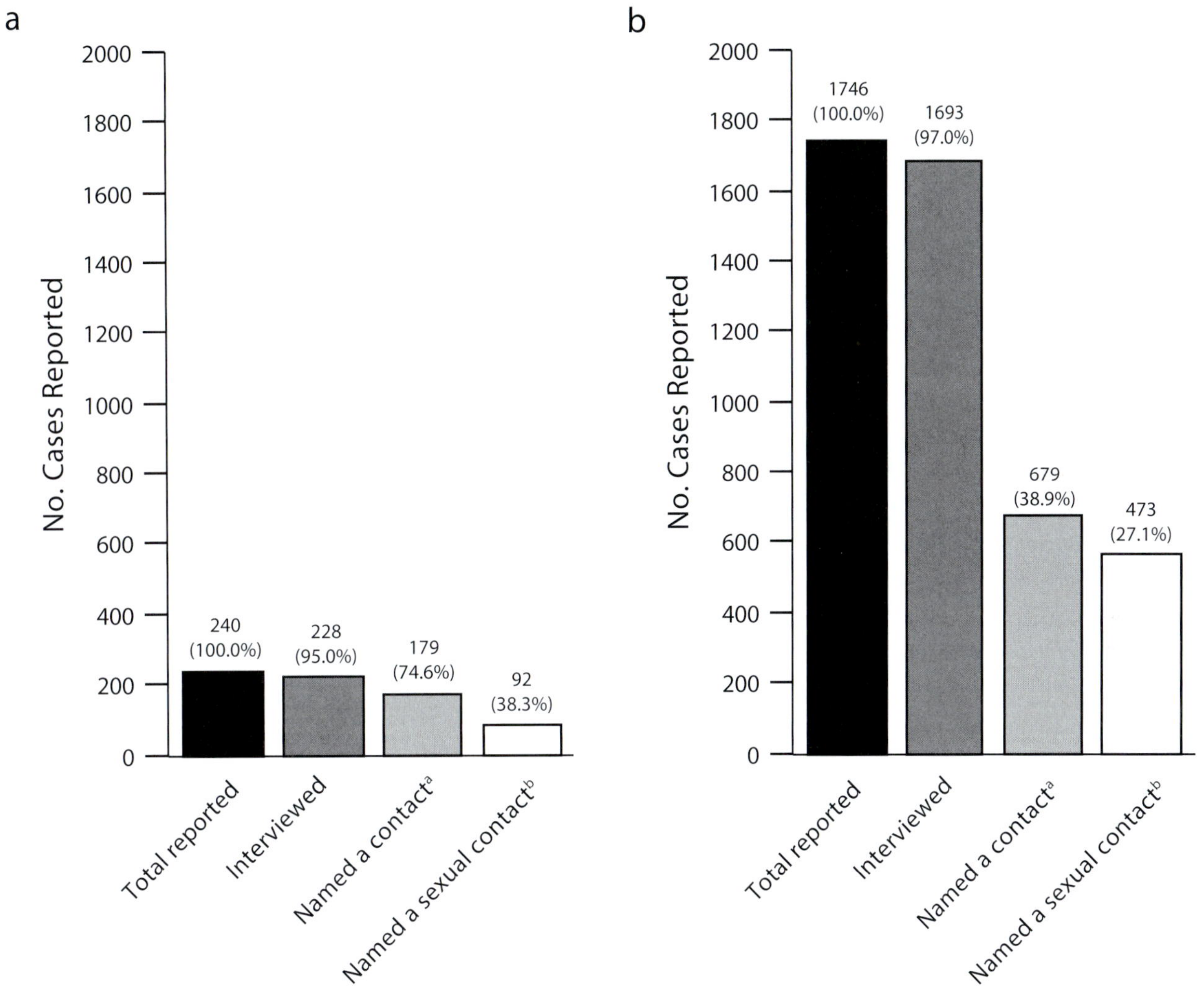

FIGURE 1— Number and Proportion of Mpox Cases Reported and Interviews Conducted Among Gay, Bisexual, and Other Men Who Have Sex With Men in (a) May 17–June 30, 2022, and (b) July 1–31, 2022: 10 US Jurisdictions

Note. The proportion's denominator is the total reported for each time period. The 10 jurisdictions were CO, DC, FL, HI, ID, MI, New York City, NC, SC, and WI.

[a]Named contact refers to a close contact in the 21 days after symptom onset for whom the interviewed patient provided sufficient contact information for the health department to initiate a contact tracing investigation.

[b]Named sexual contact refers to a named contact with whom the interviewed patient engaged in sex or close intimate contact.

MSM about ways to modify sexual behaviors to prevent mpox acquisition. A survey of MSM conducted during August 2022 found that nearly half of respondents had reduced their number of sexual partners since learning about the mpox outbreak.[11] The decrease in both the named sexual contact and unnamed contact indices in our analysis might be partially related to reductions in the number of sexual partners among MSM. The incubation period for mpox may also contribute to the observed decrease in contacts; MSM receiving a diagnosis in early July were likely exposed in June (possibly at Gay Pride Month events) and could have fewer contacts at the time of diagnosis.

The decrease in the proportion of patients who named at least 1 contact suggests that, as mpox cases began to surge, MSM may have limited their interactions with all contacts because of increased awareness of symptoms or that the interview process might have been less successful at eliciting locating information about all contacts, not just sexual contacts. Many staff conducting interviews for mpox worked in general communicable disease programs and might have lacked expertise in discussing sexual behavior.

These findings might not be generalizable to other jurisdictions or time periods. The amount and type of locating information needed to classify a contact as named and the definition used to identify MSM was determined locally and varied among jurisdictions, possibly limiting comparability.

PUBLIC HEALTH IMPLICATIONS

Contact tracing for mpox is challenging because contacts may be unreported or reported without sufficient locating information. Expansion of vaccine access from only named contacts to all persons at high risk of acquisition, increases in caseload, and behavior modification may have contributed to a decreased proportion of MSM with mpox naming contacts. Contact tracing is a resource-intensive strategy that may have benefited some, but likely did not reach most exposed persons to offer prevention services, limiting its impact. Continued promotion of other public health strategies, such as behavior change recommendations and vaccination, in addition to contact tracing, may be more effective in reducing mpox transmission among MSM. AJPH

ABOUT THE AUTHORS

Anna Barry Cope, Robert D. Kirkcaldy, Paul J. Weidle, David A. Jackson, and Kyle T. Bernstein are with the Centers for Disease Control and Prevention (CDC) Mpox Emergency Response Team, Atlanta, GA. Nicholas Laramee and Robyn Weber are with the Colorado Department of Public Health and Environment, Denver. Julia Rowse and Anil Mangla are with the District of Columbia Department of Health, Washington, DC. Brian Fox and Katharine E. Saunders are with the Florida Department of Health, Tallahassee. Kristen Taniguchi and Lauren Usagawa are with the Hawaii State Department of Health, Honolulu. Megan E. Cahill is with the Idaho Department of Health and Welfare, Boise. Pauline Harrington is with the Michigan Department of Health and Human Services, Detroit. Erin K. Ricketts and Khalil Harbi are with the North Carolina Department of Health and Human Services, Raleigh. Lenka Malec and Tingting Gu Templin are with the New York City Department of Health and Mental Hygiene, New York, NY. Dan Drociuk and Terri Hannibal are with the South Carolina Department of Health and Environmental Control, Columbia. Rachel Klos is with the Wisconsin Department of Health Services, Madison. Katharine E. Saunders, Megan E. Cahill, and Erin K. Ricketts are also with the Epidemic Intelligence Service, CDC, Atlanta.

CORRESPONDENCE

Correspondence should be sent to Anna Barry Cope, 1902 Mail Service Center, Raleigh, NC 27699-1902 (email: lnu4@cdc.gov). Reprints can be ordered at https://ajph.org by clicking the "Reprints" link.

PUBLICATION INFORMATION

Full Citation: Cope AB, Kirkcaldy RD, Weidle PJ, et al. Evaluation of public health contact tracing for mpox among gay, bisexual, and other men who have sex with men—10 US jurisdictions, May 17–July 31, 2022. *Am J Public Health*. 2023;113(7): 815–818.

Acceptance Date: March 21, 2023.

DOI: https://doi.org/10.2105/AJPH.2023.307301

CONTRIBUTORS

A. B Cope conceptualized, designed, and performed the analysis; wrote the article; and approved the final version. R. D. Kirkcaldy, P. J. Weidle, D. A. Jackson, and K. T. Bernstein conceptualized and designed the analysis, revised the article, and approved the final version. N. Laramee, R. Weber, J. Rowse, A. Mangla, B. Fox, K. E. Saunders, K. Taniguchi, L. Usagawa, M. E. Cahill, P. Harrington, E. K. Ricketts, K. Harbi, L. Malec, T. G. Templin, D. Drociuk, T. Hannibal, and R. Klos collected and contributed data, revised the article, and approved the final version.

ACKNOWLEDGMENTS

This study was supported in part by an appointment to the Applied Epidemiology Fellowship Program administered by the Council of State and Territorial Epidemiologists and funded by the CDC Cooperative Agreement 1NU38OT000297-03-00.

Note. The findings and conclusions in this report are those of the authors and do not necessarily represent the official position of the CDC.

CONFLICTS OF INTEREST

The authors report no conflicts of interest.

HUMAN PARTICIPANT PROTECTION

This activity was reviewed by the CDC and was conducted consistent with applicable federal law and CDC policy (see, e.g., 45 CFR part 46, 21 CFR part 56, 42 USC §241(d), 5 USC §552a, 44 USC §3501 et seq.). This activity was determined to be nonresearch and did not require Human Research Protection Office review.

REFERENCES

1. Minhaj FS, Ogale YP, Whitehill F, et al. Monkeypox outbreak—nine states, May 2022. *MMWR Morb Mortal Wkly Rep*. 2022;71(23):764–769. https://doi.org/10.15585/mmwr.mm7123e1
2. Centers for Disease Control and Prevention. US mpox case trends reported to CDC. Available at: https://www.cdc.gov/poxvirus/mpox/response/2022/mpx-trends.html. Accessed March 13, 2023.
3. Philpott D, Hughes CM, Alroy KA, et al. Epidemiologic and clinical characteristics of mpox cases—United States, May 17–July 22, 2022. *MMWR Morb Mortal Wkly Rep*. 2022;71(32):1018–1022. https://doi.org/10.15585/mmwr.mm7132e3
4. The White House. Fact sheet: Biden-Harris administration's mpox outbreak response. June 28, 2022. Available at: https://www.whitehouse.gov/briefing-room/statements-releases/2022/06/28/fact-sheet-biden-harris-administrations-monkeypox-outbreak-response. Accessed April 3, 2023.
5. Centers for Disease Control and Prevention. Safer sex, social gatherings, and mpox. Available at: https://www.cdc.gov/poxvirus/monkeypox/prevention/sexual-health.html. Accessed January 5, 2023.
6. Cope AB, Bernstein K, Matthias J, et al. Unnamed partners from syphilis partner services interviews, 7 jurisdictions. *Sex Transm Dis*. 2020;47(12): 811–818. https://doi.org/10.1097/OLQ.0000000000001269
7. Menza TW, De Lore JS, Fleming M, Golden MR. Partner notification for gonococcal and chlamydial infections in men who have sex with men: success is underestimated by traditional disposition codes. *Sex Transm Dis*. 2008;35(1):84–90. https://doi.org/10.1097/OLQ.0b013e31814fb125
8. Nguyen TQ, Kohn RP, Ng RC, Philip SS, Cohen SE. Historical and current trends in the epidemiology of early syphilis in San Francisco, 1955 to 2016. *Sex Transm Dis*. 2018;45(9S suppl 1):S55–S62. https://doi.org/10.1097/OLQ.0000000000000870
9. Mimiaga MJ, Reisner SL, Tetu AM, et al. Partner notification after STD and HIV exposures and infections: knowledge, attitudes, and experiences of Massachusetts men who have sex with men. *Public Health Rep*. 2009;124(1):111–119. https://doi.org/10.1177/003335490912400114
10. Brewer DD. Case-finding effectiveness of partner notification and cluster investigation for sexually transmitted diseases/HIV. *Sex Transm Dis*. 2005; 32(2):78–83. https://doi.org/10.1097/01.olq.0000153574.38764.0e
11. Delaney KP, Sanchez T, Hannah M, et al. Strategies adopted by gay, bisexual, and other men who have sex with men to prevent mpox virus transmission—United States, August 2022. *MMWR Morb Mortal Wkly Rep*. 2022;71(35): 1126–1130. https://doi.org/10.15585/mmwr.mm7135e1

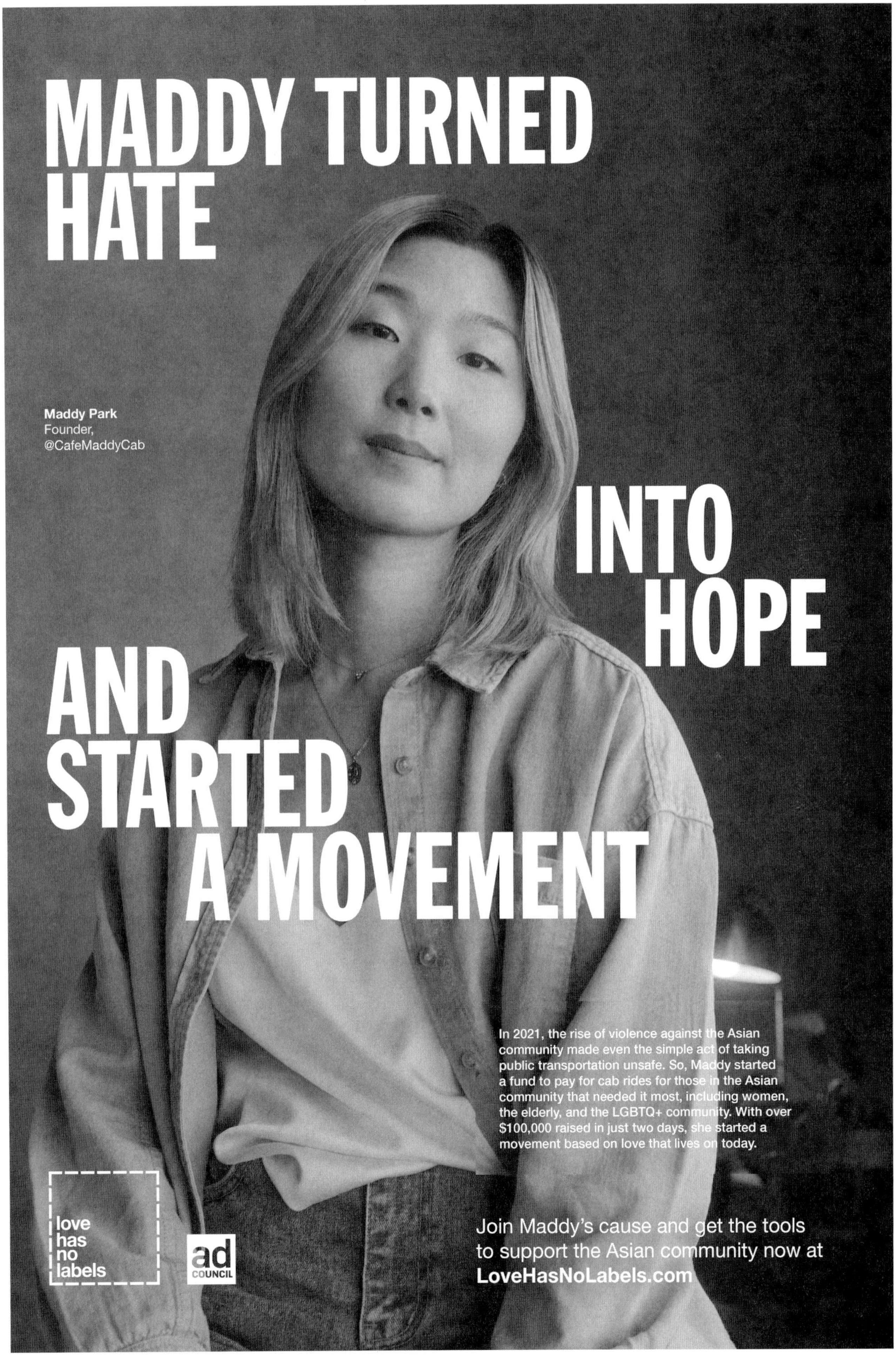

MADDY TURNED HATE
Maddy Park
Founder,
@CafeMaddyCab
INTO HOPE
AND STARTED A MOVEMENT
In 2021, the rise of violence against the Asian community made even the simple act of taking public transportation unsafe. So, Maddy started a fund to pay for cab rides for those in the Asian community that needed it most, including women, the elderly, and the LGBTQ+ community. With over $100,000 raised in just two days, she started a movement based on love that lives on today.
love has no labels
ad COUNCIL
Join Maddy's cause and get the tools to support the Asian community now at
LoveHasNoLabels.com

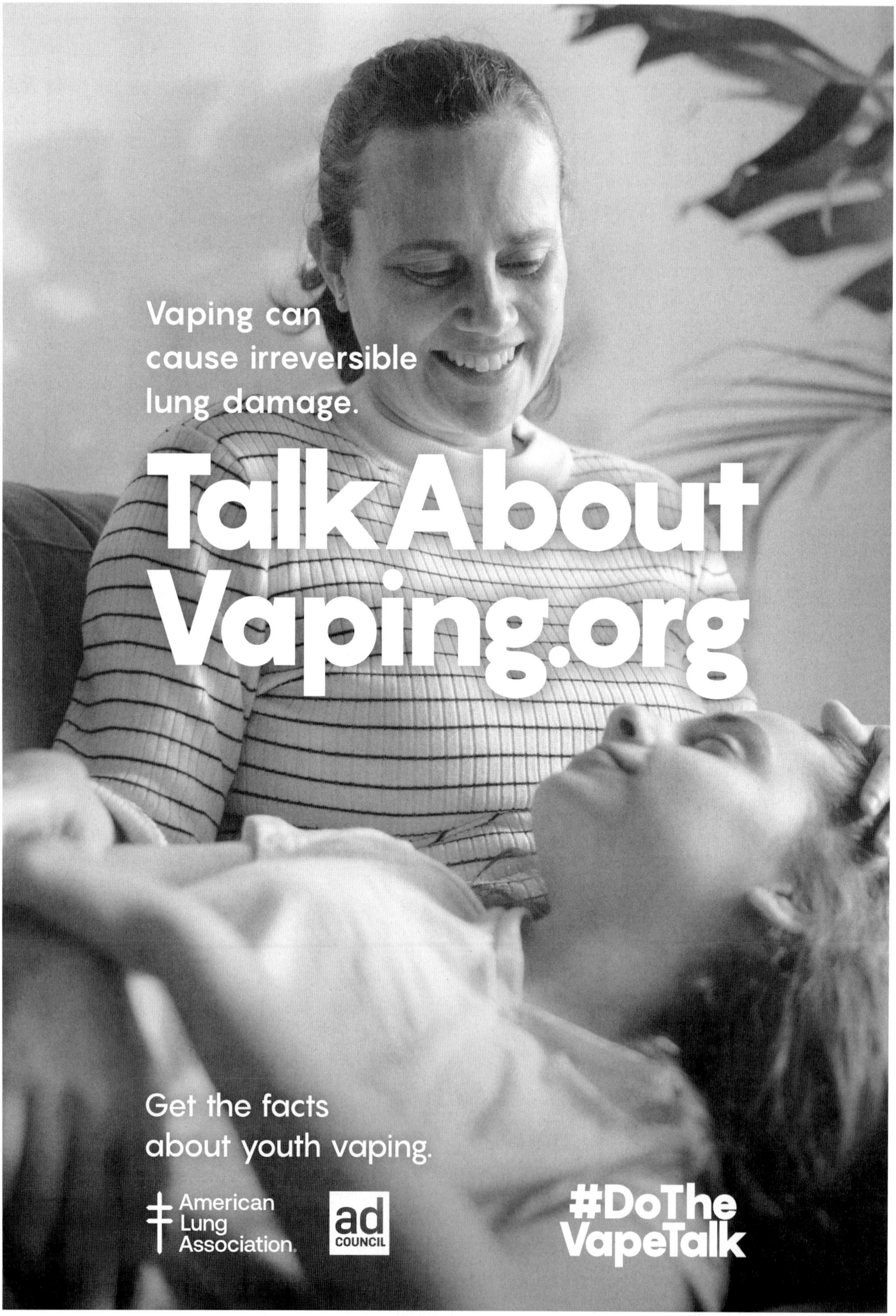

Vaping can cause irreversible lung damage.
TalkAboutVaping.org
Get the facts about youth vaping.
American Lung Association.
ad COUNCIL
#DoTheVapeTalk

GET DOWN WITH YOUR BLOOD PRESSURE™

1
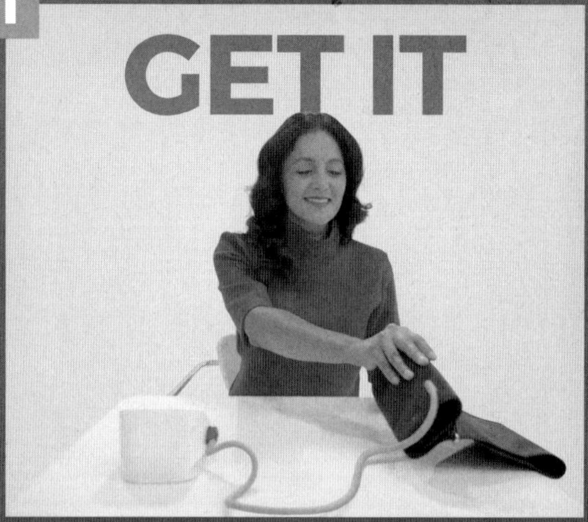

2
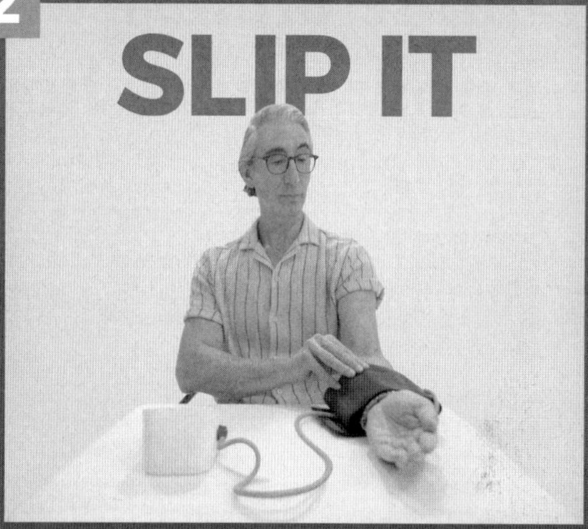

3
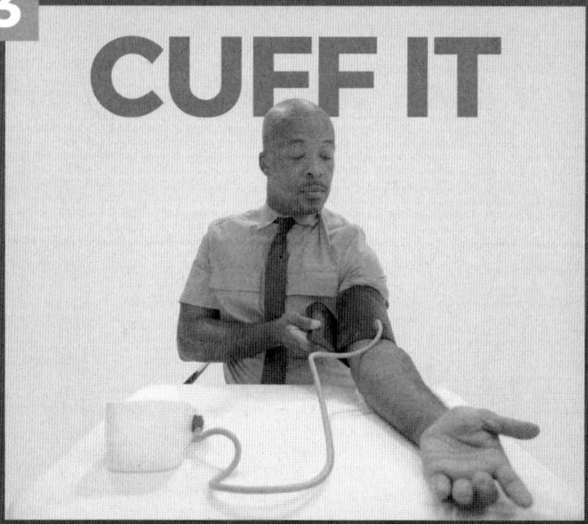

4
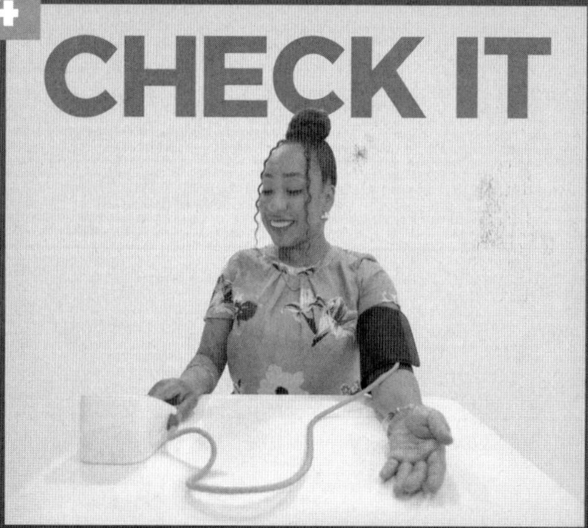

Check it every day. Self-monitoring is power.

ad COUNCIL

American Heart Association

AMA AMERICAN MEDICAL ASSOCIATION

Visit: ManageYourBP.org

Or scan code for more.

In partnership with HHS Office of Minority Health and Health Resources and Services Administration under cooperative agreements CPIMP211227 and CPIMP211228.

AdoptUSKids

ad COUNCIL

His first football season, Isaiah told us, ‘Wear a jersey with my name on it. I want everyone to know you’re here for me.’

Darnell and Denna, adopted 16-year-old Isaiah

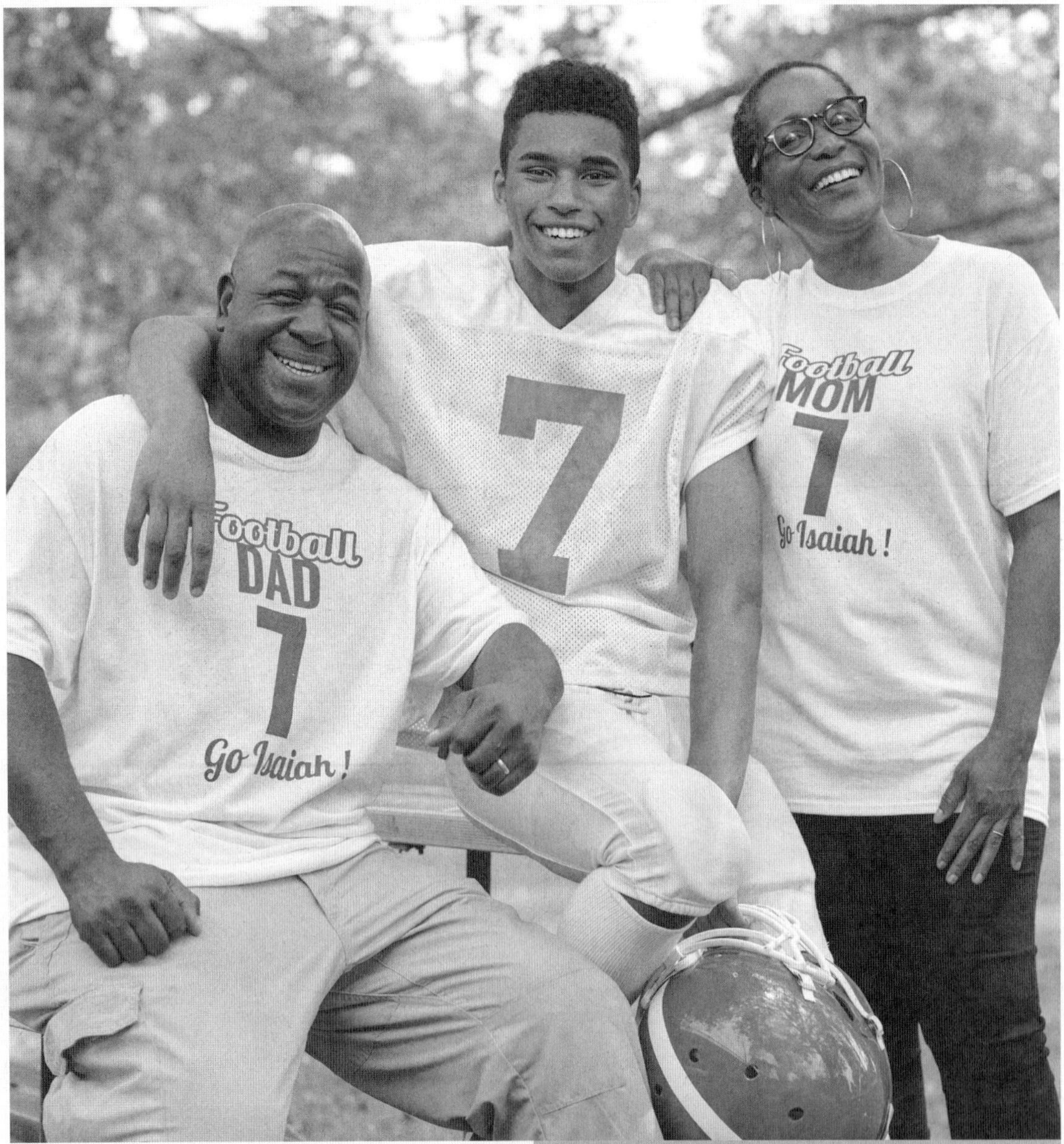

LEARN ABOUT ADOPTING A TEEN
YOU CAN’T IMAGINE THE REWARD

ADOPTUSKIDS.ORG